Neurosis: Understanding Common Mental Illness

'Psychiatry cannot advance without a good classification. We have failed to achieve this, most particularly with common mental disorders. This important book by Peter Tyrer shows a way forward, giving special attention to mixed anxiety and depressive disorders, the most important diagnosis of all. It should be mandatory reading for all psychiatrists.'

David Goldberg, Professor Emeritus, Institute of Psychiatry,
King's College London, UK

'DSM-5 & ICD-11 are splitter systems that artificially divide the diagnostic pie into tiny slices. The resulting artificial and misleading "comorbidity" often leads to fragmented and excessive treatments. Tyrer beautifully demonstrates the clinical realities that patients are necessarily more complicated than diagnostic systems and that flexible formulation is more important than rigid adherence to criteria sets. This is an extremely valuable book for all mental health professionals at all levels of training and experience.'

Allen Frances, MD, Professor and Chair Emeritus, Department of Psychiatry,
Duke University, Durham, NC, USA, and Chair, DSM-IV Task Force

'This highly readable book has long been needed. It is an essential reference for improving clinical thinking, whether you are a physician or a psychologist. It helps building unitary perspectives that may shed light on phenomena that would otherwise remain scattered in the patient's story. What is shared by syndromes such as anxiety, panic, phobic disturbances and irritability may be as important as the differences between them and conditions that are apparently comorbid could be part of the same general neurotic syndrome.'

Giovanni A. Fava, MD, Clinical Professor of Psychiatry, University at Buffalo,
State University of New York, Buffalo, NY, USA

Neurosis

Understanding Common Mental Illness

Peter Tyrer

Emeritus Professor of Community Psychiatry Imperial College of Science, Technology and Medicine, London, and Consultant in Transformation Psychiatry, Lincolnshire Partnership NHS Foundation Trust

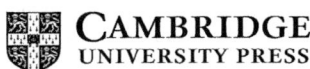

CAMBRIDGE
UNIVERSITY PRESS

CAMBRIDGE
UNIVERSITY PRESS

University Printing House, Cambridge CB2 8BS, United Kingdom

One Liberty Plaza, 20th Floor, New York, NY 10006, USA

477 Williamstown Road, Port Melbourne, VIC 3207, Australia

314–321, 3rd Floor, Plot 3, Splendor Forum, Jasola District Centre,
New Delhi – 110025, India

103 Penang Road, #05–06/07, Visioncrest Commercial, Singapore 238467

Cambridge University Press is part of the University of Cambridge.

It furthers the University's mission by disseminating knowledge in the pursuit of
education, learning, and research at the highest international levels of excellence.

www.cambridge.org
Information on this title: www.cambridge.org/9781911623656
DOI: 10.1017/9781911623823

First published 2022

Printed in the United Kingdom by TJ Books Limited, Padstow Cornwall

A catalogue record for this publication is available from the British Library.

Library of Congress Cataloging-in-Publication Data
Names: Tyrer, Peter J. author.
Title: Neurosis : understanding common mental illness / Peter Tyrer.
Description: Cambridge, United Kingdom ; New York, NY : Cambridge University Press, [2022] | Includes
bibliographical references and index.
Identifiers: LCCN 2022004173 (print) | LCCN 2022004174 (ebook) | ISBN 9781911623656 (paperback) |
ISBN 9781911623823 (ebook)
Subjects: MESH: Syndrome | Neurotic Disorders | Comorbidity | Depressive Disorder | Anxiety Disorders |
Personality Disorders | Longitudinal Studies
Classification: LCC RC346 (print) | LCC RC346 (ebook) | NLM WM 170 | DDC 616.8–dc23/eng/20220412
LC record available at https://lccn.loc.gov/2022004173
LC ebook record available at https://lccn.loc.gov/2022004174

ISBN 978-1-911-62365-6 Paperback

Dedicated to the memory of Philip Snaith (1933–2003), Senior Lecturer in Psychiatry, University of Leeds, who taught not wisely but too well

Contents

Figures

Tables

Foreword

Books that are primarily concerned with the implications of classifications of psychiatric disorders have always been less common than new classifications themselves.[1] This is unfortunate, because all classifications, including those which aspire to being 'atheoretical', embody many fundamental assumptions about the nature of their subject matter. They also have a major influence on how their users conceptualise the phenomena in question. Indeed, this may well be why new typologies appear so frequently, for those who are persuaded to adopt them will also, wittingly or unwittingly, adopt most of their authors' underlying assumptions. Treatises devoted to the classification of neuroses are particularly uncommon. It is generally assumed that the classification of psychotic disorders or of depressive illnesses is more important, and also that these topics can be more profitably discussed because more relevant empirical evidence is available. This book is therefore as unusual as it is welcome.

Dr Tyrer describes what will be for the next decade or so the two most influential and widely used classifications of neurotic disorders – the forthcoming (10th) revision of the *International Classification of Diseases* (ICD-10) and the American Psychiatric Association's classifications, DSM-III and DSM-III-R.[2] He focuses on the differences between them and the novel concepts, like panic disorder, which are common to both. He also discusses the implications of these differences and the relevant empirical evidence – the clinical trials and family studies and follow-up studies – that helps to establish the validity of the diagnostic concepts concerned. He therefore not only describes the phenomena of neurotic illness and contemporary classifications of these phenomena; he also raises important practical and theoretical questions that might otherwise have remained unasked.

Dr Tyrer writes as a practising clinician, observing as he does so, with only the faintest hint of menace, that as 'the fate of any classification depends on the reaction of its main users, it is clinicians who hold the key to success' (Tyrer, 1989, p. xi). This stance is one of this book's greatest strengths, for it is apparent in every chapter that the text has been written by someone who combines a comprehensive knowledge of the literature with extensive personal experience of the symptomatology, treatment, and prognosis of neurotic disorders. Dr Tyrer has, of course, prejudices of his own. He remains convinced that 'neurosis' is still a valuable concept, that different clinical presentations are less discrete and stable than the architects of DSM-III have assumed, that new concepts should not be adopted until they have been validated by long-term follow-up studies, and that patients with a fluctuating mélange of depressive, anxious, and obsessional symptoms are so common that the term 'general neurotic syndrome' must be retained to describe them. Several experienced psychiatrists already share these views; others will be converted to them by reading this important monograph.

R. E. Kendell
Department of Psychiatry, Edinburgh University

---

[1] This was the foreword to the precursor of this book published in 1989. It is highly relevant today. Robert Kendell died in December, 2002.
[2] The current text uses ICD-11, throughout.

Acknowledgements

This book has benefited greatly from frank comments received from colleagues. These have reduced some of my egotistical opinions and helped to create a more balanced text. Unadulterated criticism from friends is always a great leveller. In alphabetical order, I thank Gavin Andrews for our harmonious interaction about the general neurotic syndrome; Dr Barbara Barrett and Professor Sarah Byford for economic advice; Professor German Berrios and his wife, Doris, for helping me to understand Cullen's work on neurosis; Professor Patricia Casey for helping to define the position of adjustment disorders in common mental illness; Professor Kate Davidson for getting my CBT language in order; the late Sir Richard Doll for his advice about follow-up; Professor Chris Dowrick and Dr Jayati Das-Munshi for discussions about mixed anxiety and depression; Professor Sir David Goldberg for his stimulating and sometimes provocative comments about the classification of common mental disorders; the late Robert Kendell, his daughter, Kate, and his widow, Ann, for their help in understanding the purpose of diagnosis; Alan Kerr for helping me to understand the work of the 1972 Newcastle group in their publications on affective disorders; Michael King and the members of the MENCOG MRC Collaborative Research Group for their assistance in the 12-year follow-up, Phil Levy for help with illustrations; Professor Glyn Lewis for pointing out the real reasons for reluctance to diagnose anxiety and depression together, and for creating the Lewis Prediction; 'Lizzie', one of the patients in the study for her story; Professor Richard Mindham for giving me context to the Nottingham psychiatric services in the 1970s; Professor Roger Mulder for saying it like it is; NHS Digital and Sylvia Teale for their help in following up patients in the longer term; Northampton Research Ethics Committee for their understanding about cold-calling; Jessica Papworth of Cambridge University Press for guiding the book to publication; Professor Gene Paykel for constant encouragement; Dr George Stein for giving historical substance to personality disorder; the Library Services at the Royal College of Psychiatrists for helping with background material, especially the works of Adolf Meyer; and my wife, Helen, for being the most effective follow-up interview specialist on the planet.

But my greatest indebtedness is to the people who carried out the initial assessments in the study so conscientiously (Paul Barczak, Judith Brothwell, Claire Darling, Brian Ferguson, Susan Gregory, David Kingdon, Siobhan Murphy, and Nick Seivewright) and the statisticians who have helped in the analyses at all stages. Dr Tony Johnson, formerly of the MRC Biostatistics Unit in Cambridge, carried out almost all the analyses of the data from the randomised trial in 1988 to the 12-year follow-up, and who also assisted at 30 years. Professor Min Yang has been tireless in assessing and analysing the data over the whole period of follow-up and without her help this book would not have been completed. My brother, Stephen, and my son, Jonathan, were also very helpful in the early stages of the study. The full data of the study, including the anonymised data base, have been placed in the University of Nottingham Manuscripts and Special Collections, MS 1048.

Introduction

Neurosis is passé, neurosis belongs to history, neurosis is dead. So why am I writing this book? The reason is that we need to be aware of, even if we do not embrace, information that suggests the way we now look at common mental illness is not necessarily the most accurate or productive way of understanding, and more importantly, treating it. I also introduce this book with the foreword to its predecessor (Tyrer, 1989), written by the late Robert Kendell, and this also explains why I am publishing at this time. Robert, whom I will refer to as Bob from now on, was a stickler for accuracy and rarely wrote anything down that he could not defend with facts. His foreword was written 32 years ago but is just as apposite today – he actually could have written it today with the same wording, and this in itself reflects the poverty of attention that this subject has received since 1989. His statement 'new concepts should not be adopted until they have been validated by long-term follow-up studies, and the patients with a fluctuating mélange of depressive, anxious and obsessional symptoms are so common that the term "general neurotic syndrome" must be retained to describe them', is the keynote to this book. The central part of this book presents the results of a long-term follow-up study of the general neurotic syndrome, and even allowing for my prejudices (as Bob K rightly points out) it is difficult to ignore the findings that support it.

Is it appropriate to go back to the old concept of neurosis? Of course not. That is not what I am arguing, but the old concepts still offer us a level of understanding that should at least make us pause before we gallop off into the extremes of neuroscience or abandon classification altogether in favour of holistic understanding.

The arguments presented here are based on current evidence, much of it relatively new in connection with a 30-year study, and although the gaps sometimes have to be filled by opinion, I hope this will be regarded as informed and consistent, and where there are cogent alternatives, I hope they will all be acknowledged. The current notions of common mental disorders are all open to both support and criticism, but most would agree that they have not yet greatly advanced the lot of those who suffer from them.

Let us go back to some lines from three centuries ago. 'Have you no consideration for my poor nerves?' 'You mistake me, my dear. I have a high respect for your nerves. They are my old friends. I have heard you mention them with consideration these twenty years at least.'

Many people will recognise these lines immediately[1]. A Mr Bennet uttered them, deciding to respond to his neurotic wife with detached amusement rather than conflict. But therein lies his quandary. He makes no attempt to reform his wife, to alleviate her continuing 'nerves' and what are now frequently named 'medically unexplained symptoms',

---

[1] Of course, they come from Jane Austen's *Pride and Prejudice*, so well known that no reference is needed.

and when they become too much to bear, he retires to his sanctuary, The Library. He assumes, and the world will assume, that his wife, Mrs Bennet (she appears to lack a first name as in the Bennet household only the children have Christian names), will continue her merry dance with neurotic symptoms until she is released by death.

Do we look on Mrs Bennet in a completely different way now? I do not think we do. We still, at least in conversations in off-hand moments to people we feel we can trust, refer to people as 'nervous' or 'neurotic', and even though the Mrs Bennets, when seen by health professionals, often come away with a Greco-Latin epithet followed by disorder, the outcome is often not very different from that of the original Mrs Bennet. We have improved in mental health literacy so that she is no longer a figure of fun (Jane Austen could have been a little more generous here but it would have spoiled the novel), but are those who have followed her much improved in life satisfaction or personal satisfaction? It would be hard to say 'yes'.

But when you look at textbooks of psychiatry you might think very differently. Each of the disorders formerly described as neurotic are demarcated, walled off, and details given of their epidemiology, their origins, their clinical manifestations, their preferred treatment, and their outcomes. Even better, a case history can be added that encapsulates all that is pertinent to the condition. 'So here we have a classical case of social anxiety', or 'a beautiful example of panic disorder progressing to agoraphobia', or 'a paradigm of all the features of generalised anxiety disorder', but in practice the newly qualified doctor finds it very hard to identify them. Maurice Pappworth, a scourge of the medical establishment in the middle years of the last century, was a very effective teacher of medicine, and he reminded his students that their most important tasks were to observe, examine, and record what they found, rather than be a slave to texts on the subject (Pappworth, 1971). He stressed that 'classical examples' of diseases became classical because they were good for textbooks but in practice are very rare, and most diseases present in more complicated ways.

It is the same with the conditions that have followed the loss of neurosis. They look good, smell good, and seem convincing, but in practice tend to merge together, and the textbook chapters betray this when they add a section on comorbidity at the end, a subject that we will come to later on many occasions in the rest of this book. But because these new conditions have been given special status, especially since the introduction of the DSM-III in 1980, they are respectable diagnoses, and are almost always examined separately in research studies. This means that there are now very few studies in which two or more common mental illnesses are examined together as though they might represent a unity.

But to understand what has happened with neurosis in the last 300 years we need to re-enact its beginnings and its demise.

The Birth of Neurosis

The four humours of Hippocrates, black bile, yellow bile, phlegm and blood, dominated medical understanding for 3,000 years, and medical advances only came with better knowledge of anatomy, physiology, and technology right at the end of this period. Psychiatry had very little part to play in this: as we are reminded repeatedly by all who criticise the profession, mental illness very rarely leaves evidence of its presence on the structure of the body.

The period at the end of the eighteenth century is referred to as the Scottish Enlightenment, when, following the example of the philosopher David Hume, every aspect of knowledge was questioned and re-examined, and so it was not surprising that mental illness came under the focus of enlightenment too and was followed by others. 'Neurosis' became the new word for common mental illness. It was first formulated as 'nervous diseases' by Robert Whytt (1765) to 'describe the common features of the disorders which are the subject of the following observations . . . under the name of flatulent, spasmodic, hypochondriac or hysteric'. Whytt was an experimenter too and attempted to find pathological differences in his patients. This, not surprisingly, led him up the blind alley of reductionism. His investigations suggesting the nerves of women were more motile than those of men and so predisposed them to neurosis, fell flat.

His successor as Professor of the Practice of Medicine at Edinburgh University, William Cullen, was not primarily a researcher but a synthesiser. He organised the writings of Whytt more coherently and described neuroses as a unitary group of nervous disorders (Cullen, 1777) with a much wider focus than the concept subsequently possessed, but included depression, anxiety, hysteria, and hypochondriasis. This was new. Although hypochondriasis and hysteria were described in earlier texts from Theophrastus onwards, they were only brought together by Cullen. Piñero also gives particular credit to Thomas Willis and Thomas Sydenham in their writings a century earlier in clarifying earlier definitions (Piñero, 1983, pp. 2–4) of hypochondriasis and hysteria in advance of Cullen. When two or more disorders represent two aspects of the same disorder the word 'consanguinity' is more appropriate than co-occurrence or comorbidity (Tyrer, 1996) and the diligent Scottish investigators were the first to join this range of disorders together as a consanguineous condition.

In a curious paradox, just as Robert Spitzer destroyed the concept of neurosis in the DSM-III by harnessing groups of experts and creating consensuses to split neurosis, William Cullen did the same in harnessing all the terms for nervousness and linking them. Both men planned in the same way. Cullen thought of the neuroses in the same way as the stellar classifier of the day, Carl Linnaeus, as genera and species. The four genera were the comas (species: apoplexy and paralysis – including hysterical paralysis); adynamiae (species: dyspepsia, hypochondriasis, and chlorosis – a nervous disease of blood-forming organs [cf. anaemia]); spasmi (species: tetanus, trismus, epilepsy, palpitations, colic, hysteria); and vesaniae (species: melancholia, mania, somnolence). Cullen's followers expanded and modified this list in subsequent decades, and although the neuroses are included here, the full classification looks very much like an early edition of DSM-III, but with each condition spared the epithet of the ubiquitous noun 'disorder'.

Because the Scottish Enlightenment led the way in European science the works of Whytt and Cullen became widely known across the continent and were quickly translated into other languages. In retrospect they probably had more traction and popularity in Europe as a whole than in England, where the Enlightenment was not looked on with universal approval.

The Recognition of Personality Status in Neurosis

Adolf Meyer (1866–1950) is now almost totally forgotten as a psychiatric innovator. This is curious as he was the pre-eminent figure in American psychiatry in the first half of the twentieth century. This is partly because he was one of the few people who could bridge the gap between the Kraepelinian search for meaningful diagnoses similar to those in medicine, and the psychoanalytical school, who generally abhorred diagnosis as an unwelcome interloper interfering in the real enquiry, the search for psychiatric meaning. One of the reasons he is not remembered is that his writings are almost indecipherable. Meyer was born in Swiss Germany and although he mastered English well when it came to lecturing, he seemed to view the written page as a place where there was competition to write the longest and most impenetrable sentences.

This is a pity, as he had some important observations to make. He could be regarded as the originator of 'whole person medicine'. He is best known for the emphasis he makes on getting to know patients properly before deciding how to help them. This may seem an unnecessary aphorism now but it certainly wasn't in 1902 when he wrote, 'we need a crusade against empty utterances of opinion when facts are available, against the use of diagnostic terms which have no definite meaning' (Meyer 1902, p. 101). Bob Kendell, in his masterly book, *The Role of Diagnosis in Psychiatry*, noted that most psychiatrists, whether in training or very experienced, reach their final diagnosis within a few minutes of an interview (Kendell, 1975a). You could regard this as an efficient diagnostic system but if the wrong decision is made prematurely the outcome can be disastrous.

Meyer would have been heavily critical of diagnostic guidelines (especially easily learned operational criteria) that dominate current assessment because he rightly felt that attaching a diagnosis could deflect interest about other important elements that were not included in that diagnosis. At worst, the person becomes a diagnosis and loses individuality.

But the real reason I am giving attention to Adolf Meyer is that he gave more attention to personality status than all his predecessors and most of those who followed him. He felt very strongly that without the assessment of personality the mental state examination was incomplete. Many people consider that he went too far in emphasising the uniqueness of the individual and their personality, but he made sure that everyone knew his views. He argued that psychiatric disorders were reactions of the person to events – you could call this the beginning of life-events research – and as each person had limited ways of reacting, these 'reaction types' could be used to delineate psychiatric disorders. These ideas were adopted more strongly in the United Kingdom than in the Americas, and one of the most popular mental health textbooks of all time, Henderson and Gillespie's *Textbook of Psychiatry*, first published in 1927 and extending to a tenth edition by 1969, used Meyer's concepts throughout.

It is sad that Meyer did not develop his ideas further with respect to personality. Nonetheless, he felt the subject was extremely important and insisted on teaching it himself when his colleagues proved to be inadequate in getting the message across to students. His textbook pronouncements became lost in the verbal thicket but in his teaching he was very persuasive and convincing, and even this comes through when he writes about personality.

In my training of medical students, I have each student work out a fairly systematic personality study of the worker himself or herself and a more summary sketch of a few outstanding contrasting classmates or known persons. (Meyer, 1902, p. 247)

For this reason each student is asked to make a study of a specific person, preferably of himself, together with comparisons with three classmates showing particularly outstanding contrasts and differences. Our study deals with the concrete objective and not really introspective performances, the methods of their presentation and formulation, and the testing and using of the data and problems of adjustment of a personality. (p. 259)

He gave them tests, asking to what extent satisfaction was determined by performance and mood, capacity, opportunity and ambition, and the need to be appreciated by others. He maintained that every medical practitioner should assess the 'person and attending personality' whenever they assessed a patient.

Where Meyer went off the rails was in setting up a system of classification emphasising that everything that impacted on the 'oneness' of the person was a reaction to the genetic, developmental, and environmental factors that made that person unique. He called these reactions the 'ergasias', and this word was translated by others into 'reaction types' in place of psychiatric diagnoses. So, his followers, eventually more outside the United States than within it, used this phrase repeatedly between 1925 and 1960. This included the 10th edition of Henderson and Gillespie's frequently edited textbook (Henderson and Batchelor, 1969), the most interesting parts of which are the case histories, which are not only described in great detail but are clearly authentic, not airbrushed into matched diagnoses like the ones Pappworth so disparaged. It is interesting how Henderson established the accuracy of his case accounts. Morrison (2016) describes how he established routine 'staff meetings' at Gartnavel Hospital in Glasgow in which a psychiatrist asked questions of a patient and a stenographer in the room recorded word-for-word the conversation that passed between the two parties. Henderson was following his mentor, Adolf Meyer, identifying the person clearly before making any judgement about diagnosis.

Why didn't Meyer go further and attempt to tease out the personality component of his diagnostic system? Nobody knows, but by concentrating on the 'ergasias', a term nobody ever used in practice, he lost the support of those who might otherwise have taken his views forward more systematically.

Neurosis and Neuroticism

What is surprising is that so few people have made any sort of diagnostic connection between neurosis and neuroticism. The terms have just melded together without their implications being considered. It is this relationship that led me to suggest the existence of the general neurotic syndrome in the 1980s and led to the book published late in the decade (Tyrer, 1989).

The central argument was a simple one. If so many common mental illnesses are linked to neuroticism in the form of a personality variable, might it not be that the mental disorders from which they suffer are also linked to neuroticism to the extent that they form a common group of disorders. Time after time in the 1980s, when I was writing to general practitioners about my assessment of patients in the clinic, I had to write sentences such as 'according to current classification this patient has an episode of depression but this only explains a tiny part of the clinical picture. I would regard the patient as having a mixed neurotic disorder with both anxiety and depressive symptoms with a degree of social phobia that could easily progress to agoraphobia.'

I will illustrate this, as I will repeatedly throughout this book, by describing a patient who has long-term generalised anxiety, other mood disturbance, and hypochondriasis. Yes, here she is again. She is Mrs Bennet from *Pride and Prejudice*, and as she is fictitious, she cannot take offence, and, indeed, so much will her assets impress you over the course of her evaluation, that at the end she may be proud of her diagnosis. Yes, as you might expect, I am going to argue that she exemplifies the general neurotic syndrome.

It may seem odd that Jane Austen, despite her excellent powers of observation and understanding, describes Mrs Bennet's symptoms as though they were entirely made up, or *factitious* in current parlance (whoever thought up this word with only one letter different from 'fictitious' deserves to be arraigned for language offences). So Jane describes Mrs Bennet as 'a woman of mean understanding, little information and uncertain temper', following it up by the crushing statement 'when she was discontented she fancied herself nervous'. But as every psychiatrist and general practitioner knows, Mrs Bennet is not faking her symptoms. Mr Bennet knows this too. She doesn't fancy herself nervous; she has always been nervous. When she accuses her husband of having no respect for her nerves, he again crushes her with his comments about her nerves being his old friends. And while Austen implies artifice in the words 'when she was discontented she fancied herself nervous', she is really telling us, very clearly, that Mrs Bennet has both depressive and anxious symptoms.

But, to maintain the comedy, Jane Austen will not let Mrs Bennet off the hook of ridicule. So when Elizabeth rejects the odious advances of Mr Collins, Mrs Bennet is beside herself, and clearly beside everybody else too, in her protestations of suffering:

'Not that I have much pleasure indeed in talking to anybody. People who suffer as I do from nervous complaints can have no great inclination for talking. Nobody can tell what I suffer! – But it is always so. Those who do not complain are never pitied.'

Of course, she complains over and over again about her symptoms and suffering, so we snigger into our hands at the thought that she suffers in silence. Nobody is spared the expression of her distress;

'Don't keep coughing so, Kitty, for Heaven's sake! Have a little compassion on my nerves. You tear them to pieces.'
'Nobody is on my side, nobody takes part with me, I am cruelly used, nobody feels for my poor nerves.'

What is also clear is that the physical symptoms she experiences are those of pathological anxiety; they could in no way be factitious:

'I am frightened out of my wits; and have such tremblings, such flutterings, all over me, such spasms in my side, and pains in my head, and such beatings at heart, that I can get no rest by night nor by day.'

In case you get the idea that I am over-preoccupied with Mrs Bennet, I need to state the reasons why I am dwelling on her to such an extent. It is because she is now so well known that she has become a real person, a celebrity, but is being remembered for the wrong reasons, as a target of mirth and derision, who is manipulating her symptoms to get attention for herself and has no concern for anybody else.

But this is the opposite of the truth. Mrs Bennet is the only clear-headed member of the Bennet household and she illustrates the evolutionary benefit of the general neurotic syndrome, developed in more detail in the last chapter of this book. At the family home in Longbourn, her husband has opted out of all responsibility; her eldest daughter, Jane, is besotted and cannot think straight; Elizabeth, on whom we now all dote, is pursuing an idealistic path in life with no consideration of nineteenth century realpolitik; and the three other daughters are just capricious and silly. Only Mrs Bennet has the understanding, the drive, and the foresight to ensure that the estate stays in the family.

I hope your interest has been stimulated. But now we need to formulate the general neurotic syndrome in more detail, knowing that Mrs Bennet will be looking over my shoulder to make sure I do not err.

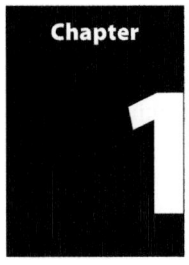

Chapter

1

The General Neurotic Syndrome

As this book is primarily about the general neurotic syndrome (GNS), I need to be convincing in creating the groundwork to persuade the reader to continue to read. Some may feel this syndrome is a fictitious creation and so I will have to work even harder to persuade these sceptics; all I would ask at this point is for people to have an open mind. The general neurotic syndrome is not (yet) a familiar term, even though it should be. As it has been a subject I have had in my head for over 45 years – I hope not as an obsession but as a guiding light – I need to put my thinking about it into context.

1.1 Initial ideas

In the 1970s, when I was working in Southampton as a senior lecturer, my view of the general neurotic syndrome was very simple: 'If a person has both anxiety and depressive symptoms and some personality disturbance, the diagnosis of the general neurotic syndrome is the best way of defining the problem.' At this stage I was not certain how to define anxiety or depression or the exact nature of the personality disturbance. In defining it in this way I was also aware from my clinical practice that people with this syndrome tended to have poor outcomes.

This was a fairly limited definition, or rather an initial hypothesis that needed testing, and at the time I was not thinking of other disorders within the neurotic spectrum. Many people had theories about these and were prolix in expressing them. Alfred Adler, the well-known psychoanalyst, described most mental disorders as related to the desire to exercise power and overcome inferiority. He dwelt on this subject in writing about the 'neurotic constitution', an escape from the failure to become powerful. The neurotic symptoms each had a significant personal meaning for the patient; they became fictionalised and detached from reality (Adler, 1921). This led to the idea of a unified neurotic syndrome ('Die Einheitsneurose') but was not developed further and never really embraced in classification.

At this time, the view of 'neurosis' as an entity in clinical practice was an inchoate one in my mind. At its simplest level, it was manifest as a split between disorders in which common understandable symptoms are excessive but grounded in reality (neurosis) and those where bizarre inexplicable symptoms and behaviour are divorced from reality (psychoses). My view at this time conformed to this general idea but with the addendum that core neurosis was linked to personality.

But this was thrown into debate by what is now commonly called the Newcastle Group, a research mix of academics and clinicians together with a statistician, Roger Garside, who claimed that the common disorders of anxiety and depression could be separated using appropriate statistical methodology, and that clinicians should be able to make a primary diagnosis of anxiety or depression, with no need for both (Gurney et al., 1972; Roth et al.,

1972). The authors were unequivocal in their conclusions: 'the first component extracted from a principal components analysis of the data was bipolar, with anxiety symptoms at one pole and depressive symptoms at the other; maladaptive personality traits were mainly associated with anxiety symptoms. This finding confirms that within an affective material there are two distinct syndromes corresponding to anxiety and depression' (Roth et al., 1972, p. 158). And again, 'using discriminant function analysis the bimodality of the patients' scores (i.e., clear separation between groups) indicated that there were two distinct groups, which, moreover, corresponded closely to the clinical differentiation into anxiety state and depressive illness, thereby confirming the hypothesis' (Gurney et al., 1972, p. 165).

But did these findings tell us that anxiety and depression were separate disorders? No. Anxiety and depression were identifiable as distinct entities but were they distinguishable in practice and did this have clinical meaning? Was the evidence of separation just a statistical method to separate symptoms but not patients? There has been debate about this ever since, increasingly unsupportive of this notion over the years. Perhaps the most economical summary was Dobson's, who made a full review of the literature and ended with a delphic summary. 'The distinction' between anxiety and depression 'may be more conceptually satisfying than empirically demonstrated' (Dobson, 1985).

But there is no doubt the Newcastle Group had stirred the neurosis pot from its position of quiet somnolence. Discussions about the anxiety/depression distinction and its value in selecting treatment (Kerr et al., 1972; Schapira et al., 1972) became very common in clinical practice. I recall arguments at ward rounds in Knowle Hospital near Fareham in Hampshire; vigorous discussions where junior colleagues were castigated for not committing themselves to a single diagnosis in a patient who had both symptoms of anxiety and depression. Sometimes the argument that as personality disturbance had been described in the presentation of the case this showed the diagnosis must be an anxiety one, 'as Professor Roth has said so'.

My own view of the work of the Newcastle Group, given nearly 50 years of reflection, is that it was rather like shining a light into a dark corner for the first time. You are not quite sure what you are seeing but you carefully sketch what you can and report back. But you know you are missing a lot. It was a pity that the Newcastle Group's study only included inpatients (most patients with primary anxiety disorders rarely go into hospital) and did not test their hypotheses with another equivalent group of patients. They were also using statistical approaches that were relatively new to psychiatry but not fully understood, and in retrospect should not have been relied on to justify their arguments.

And what was the real purpose of the study? The exercise seemed almost like comparing two kinds of eating apples such as Worcester Pearmain and Cox's Orange Pippin. Visual examination reveals consistent differences between the two types of apple but when you take the broader picture the two apples are virtually identical. They come from a similar looking tree, belong to the same botanical species, and have very similar textures and flavours. Of course, it is possible to separate one from the other using the highly discriminant analysis of observation and so the two types of apple can be separated into different baskets and sold at different prices, but the fact remains they are eating apples with many more similarities than differences.

During this period I had also been involved in comparing the effectiveness of day hospitals and outpatient clinics for the treatment of anxious, phobic, and depressed patients (Tyrer & Remington, 1979; Tyrer et al., 1987). Our findings in these studies showed consistency of phobic symptoms but great inconsistency of anxiety and depressive ones over a two-year period. This reinforced the notion that the universal separation of anxiety and depression was not a useful clinical practice.

It is reasonable to ask why this subject seemed so important to me at that time, as some might find the whole issue esoteric. I had been trained in medicine and had completed higher training in the subject and had always felt that diagnosis was a very important medical task – one that could only be taken on by a doctor at that time. If the most common conditions in mental health could not be properly diagnosed, what hope was there for psychiatry? (This, of course, was at a time when diagnosis was considered a critical part of psychiatric practice; the doubts that are being expressed today hardly existed at that time.) I do not want to give the impression I was moving towards a catastrophe in my thinking but the subject had to be addressed if I was to feel confident as a practitioner.

1.2 Later Stage (1980s)

A more coherent formulation of my view of the general neurotic syndrome was made in the early 1980s, but it was created as part of a concept not too different from 'Die Einheitsneurose'. In 1985, I wrote a paper on the subject in the *Lancet*. The Lancet always prides itself on being at the beginning of a medical story and also being there at the end, but not caring about what is in between, so they were very generous in publishing this paper before anyone else had mentioned the general neurotic syndrome, which to many others must have sounded bizarre. In this paper I wrote:

> It is more appropriate to regard many of these conditions (i.e., neuroses) as manifestations of one disorder, which may be termed the 'general neurotic syndrome'. To qualify for this diagnosis patients should show at least three of the following features:
>
> (a) two or more of the following symptomatic diagnoses are present together, either now or at times in the past: agoraphobia and social phobias, panic disorder, non-psychotic depression, anxiety, and hypochondriasis (including somatoform disorders);
> (b) at least one episode of illness has developed in the absence of major stress;
> (c) There are abnormal personality features of a passive dependent or an anankastic type;
> (d) There is a history of a similar syndrome in first-degree relatives. (Tyrer, 1985)

I also added: 'these symptoms can be placed in a "handicap hierarchy" depending on the degree of social impairment for the symptoms produced'. This was accompanied by a figure of concentric circles showing the different disorders with the outer ones showing the greater handicap (Figure 1). (Because 'handicap' is now felt to be pejorative it could be replaced with disability). Thus, generalised anxiety, which is associated with the least degree of social impairment, occupies less space than the other syndromes, and agoraphobia, social phobia and hypochondriasis occupies a larger space. But I was careful to emphasise that this was not a diagnostic hierarchy; it was merely to illustrate that there was more social impairment in the outer rings.

My justification of each of these four elements follows, and here I am updating and adding to my arguments, but not changing them in any fundamental way.

1 Simultaneous and Past Presentation of Two or More Symptoms of Six Conditions

I chose these six: agoraphobia, social phobia, panic disorder, non-psychotic depression, anxiety, and hypochondriasis (including somatoform disorders), as they are the most prevalent conditions in the neurotic group. At the time of writing in 1985 there was already much evidence that there was overlap between all these disorders. This was explained in different ways:

(a) there is a hierarchy of symptomatology (Boyd et al., 1984, Coryell et al., 1988);

(b) they are a common group of disorders (Aronson, 1987);

(c) although the symptoms appear to overlap they are genuinely separate and successful intervention demonstrates their distinctiveness (e.g., pharmacological dissection, Klein, 1964, 1981).

2 The Triggering Effect of Stress

The requirement that at least 'one episode of illness has developed in the absence of major stress' was included to illustrate the importance of life events in creating mood disorders (Figure 1.1), as well as the relevance of what became known as adjustment disorders. But I specified the absence of major stress to exclude post-traumatic stress disorder, a completely separate condition, but left the option open for minor stresses at home, at work, and in relationships, to create a stepwise increment in symptoms.

So, when Mrs Bennet says to her daughter, 'Don't keep coughing so, Kitty, for Heaven's sake! Have a little compassion on my nerves. You tear them to pieces', she is illustrating the consequences of minor stress in creating symptoms, stresses which for the average person would go unnoticed. Here again personality is involved. Some years ago (Tyrer, 2007), I suggested the term 'personality diathesis' was a better one than personality disorder as the possession of such a vulnerability was a lifelong one that lowered the threshold to stress. I still think this is a better term than 'disorder' but as disorder is applied universally to all mental health conditions, we have to accept the common parlance (but see Chapter 8 for its implications).

3 There Are Abnormal Personality Features of a Passive Dependent or an Anankastic Type

I have to admit this was a partial guess at the time, but in retrospect it is justified. The reason for the choice of these two personality features emanated from a study of neurotic patients who also had a personality disorder (Tyrer, Casey & Gall, 1983). We found that anankastic and passive-dependent personality traits were most often found in those with neurotic disorder.

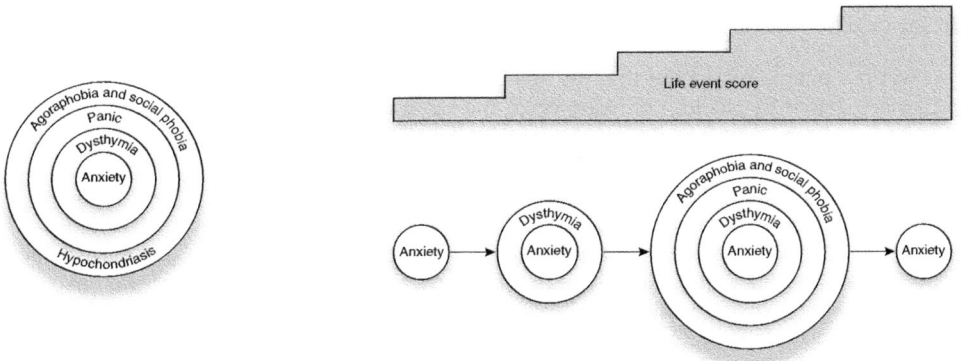

Figure 1.1 The initial formulation of the general neurotic syndrome and its components, including its variation over time in response to stresses
(From Tyrer, 1985, with kind permission of the publishers of the *Lancet*)

The simultaneous presence of a clinical syndrome (cothymia) and personality disorder might best be described as a Galenic syndrome. Galen, in his 192 AD commentary, *De Temperamentis*, described how the four (personality) humours, melancholic, sanguine, choleric, and phlegmatic, were associated with specific diseases. His four humours dominated medicine for the next 1,500 years, accompanied by the dictum that too much of one humour led to disease. The sanguine person could accumulate too much blood and so needed leeches to reduce it, the phlegmatic person with lung disease created too much phlegm, and the choleric patient needed a purgative to remove an excess of bile.

Although Galen clearly had no good knowledge of the nature of bodily diseases, his linking of personality to them was novel and needs to be resurrected in modern psychiatry. A Galenic syndrome can therefore be defined as 'a combination of personality disorder and clinical symptom complex so frequently associated that the two conditions should be considered as a single disorder'.

4 History of a Similar Syndrome in First-Degree Relatives

This is a clear reference to the genetic elements of neurotic disorder, a subject that has attracted much attention. There is unequivocal evidence that there is a genetic contribution to all the disorders within the neurotic spectrum. There is much less agreement about the role of the family environment in causation. In the words of a recent meta-analytical review: 'Panic disorder, generalized anxiety disorder, phobias, and obsessive-compulsive disorder all have significant familial aggregation. For panic disorder, generalized anxiety disorder, and probably phobias, genes largely explain this familial aggregation; the role of family environment in generalized anxiety disorder is uncertain' (Hettema et al., 2001, p. 1568).

In the case of generalised anxiety, the hypothesis that an anxious mother can create an anxious child is a very persuasive one. Behavioural psychologists call this 'modelling'; the child observes the mother (sometimes the father) showing anxious avoidance and imitates it, is also often then taught to show anxious avoidance, and, hey presto, you have an anxious child who grows up to be an anxious adult. But the data do not give strong evidence in favour of this. One of the most influential researchers in the area, Roy Plomin, asked this question in 1987: 'why are children in the same family so different from one another?' (Plomin & Daniels, 1987). Twenty-four years later he admitted he did not have an answer. He summarises his dilemma clearly:

> It was reasonable to assume that the key influences on children's development are those that are shared by children growing up in the same family: their parents' personality and family experiences, the quality of their parents' marital relationship, their parents' educational background and socioeconomic status, the neighbourhood in which they are raised and their parents' attitude to school or to discipline. Yet to the extent that these influences are shared environmentally, they cannot account for individual differences in children's development because the *salient environmental influences are non-shared* [my italics]. The message is not that family experiences are unimportant but rather that the relevant experiences are specific to each child in the family, not general to all children in the family. (Plomin, 2011)

This is a subject highly relevant to the treatment called *nidotherapy* (Tyrer, 2009) that became a subject of particular interest in the Nottingham Study, and this will appear again in this book.

1.3 Progress in Understanding the General Neurotic Syndrome since 1985

In a book I wrote in 1989, I formalised the definition of the general neurotic syndrome in the following words:

> The general neurotic syndrome is characterised by the simultaneous presence of various anxiety and depressive symptoms occurring in the absence of major psychological or physical trauma in individuals who have inhibited or dependent personalities. The diagnosis is made through a three-stage process:
>
> (1) Identification of the co-occurrence of anxiety and depressive symptoms in the absence of severe depressive illness or another significant psychiatric disorder;
> (2) Examination of environmental evidence of the symptoms and measurements of their severity;
> (3) Determination of the premorbid personality of the subject.
>
> (Tyrer, 1989, p. 154)

I also created the General Neurotic Syndrome Scale (Table 1.1)

This scale has deficiencies – not least that it was not formally tested – but the central elements are ones that I still think after a gap of 23 years are relevant to the diagnosis. I also

Table 1.1 The General Neurotic Syndrome Scale (GNSS)

Positive characteristics	Score	Negative characteristics	Score
Simultaneous presence of syndromal anxiety and depressive disorders (cothymia)	+2	Persistent phobic and obsessional symptoms	−2
Variation in the primacy of depressive and anxiety symptoms at different times	+3	Symptoms of anxiety and depression only occur in response to immediate life events	−3
If symptoms of panic, obsessive compulsive disorder, and hypochondriasis are present they do not last longer than three months	+1		
Premorbid anxious or dependent personality disorder	+3		
Premorbid anankastic (obsessive-compulsive) personality disorder	+1	Premorbid impulsive, borderline or antisocial personality disorder	−3
At least one parent has mixed anxiety depressive syndrome (cothymia)	+2		
TOTAL SCORE (no general neurotic syndrome)			0–3
TOTAL SCORE (likely general neurotic syndrome)			4–5
TOTAL SCORE (definite general neurotic syndrome)			≥ 6

excluded phobic and obsessional symptoms by giving them a minus score, and some (that now includes me) would regard a negative score as inappropriate as these conditions, as suggested in my 1985 paper, could be regarded as extensions of the syndrome. On the other hand, the better definition and consistency of phobic and obsessional symptoms can make these conditions more amenable to diagnosis. The score needed to attribute the diagnosis of the general neurotic syndrome has not changed but now I feel more strongly that the higher score of 6 is the best threshold and that a GNS score of 4 only makes the diagnosis suspect. (In the rest of the book both versions of the GNS will often appear; this is of value in showing the linear transition of what is clearly a dimensional scale.

One important advantage of the general neurotic syndrome as a diagnosis is that it does not depend on time lines. The formal classifications of the neurotic group of disorders at that time had conditions varying from a few hours (acute stress reaction) to several years (dysthymic disorder) (Figure 1.2), which really made it impossible to make clear decisions when assessing a patient for the first time. All the requirements for making the diagnosis of the general neurotic syndrome are immediately clear in the scale; the examination of present symptoms and their precipitants (if any) are all that is needed.

One of the great sources of resistance that has prevented acceptance of the general neurotic syndrome is the antipathy to joining anxiety and depression together as a single diagnosis. It is difficult to know why the resistance has been so strong. David Goldberg set the scene many years ago when he and colleagues produced the first standardised interview schedule for common mental disorders (Goldberg et al., 1970). In the second part of the schedule, the nine most common symptoms of mental illness are listed: I have placed them in Table 1.2 in terms of the most prominent mood associated with each.

I am sure everybody looking at this table will agree the overlap between anxiety and depression is massive and cannot be ignored in any sensible classification.

The schedule described by Goldberg et al. (1970), 12 years later changed its name to the Clinical Interview Schedule (Lewis, 1992). The major symptoms were the same as in 1970 but

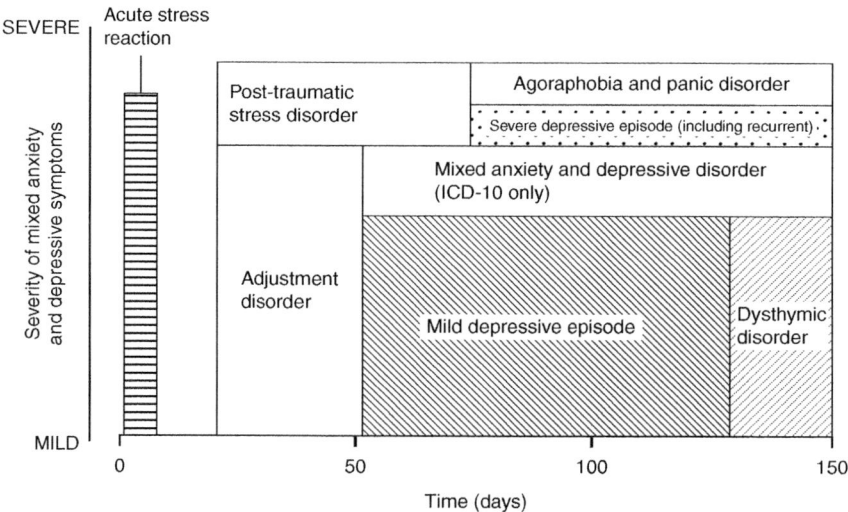

Figure 1.2 The confusing relationship between duration of symptoms and diagnosis in DSM-III and ICD-10

Table 1.2 The association of depression and anxiety with the symptoms of common mental illness

Nature of symptom	Associated mood
Somatic symptoms	anxiety and depression
Fatigue	anxiety and depression
Sleep disturbance	anxiety and depression
Irritability	anxiety and depression
Lack of concentration	anxiety and depression
Depression	depression
Anxiety and worry	anxiety
Phobias	anxiety
Obsessions and compulsions	anxiety and depression

had two more added – worry about physical health (which might now be called hypochondriasis or health anxiety) and depressive ideas – and all of these were rated reliably. The first addition was understandable and a clear omission from the first schedule. The section on depression was split into frequency and severity of depression (depression per se) and related symptoms of depression such as hopelessness and guilt (depressive ideas) (Lewis, personal communication, 2021). With so many mixed symptoms, it was therefore not at all surprising that mixed anxiety and depression became an important feature in the responses. Still, only the revised Clinical Interview Schedule (CIS-R) reported this finding; no other scales addressed it. Its importance to public health was highlighted by Das-Munshi et al. (2008) who found, through analysis of data from the National Psychiatric Morbidity surveys, the one-month prevalence of Mixed Anxiety and Depressive Disorder (MADD, a very unfortunate acronym) was 8.8 per cent and accounted for 20 per cent of all days off work in the population.

The authors made a strong case for including mixed anxiety and depression in epidemiological surveys as this condition was also associated strongly with health-related quality of life. They concluded, 'our findings strongly support the inclusion of a dimensional perspective, without which the population burden of psychological morbidity is markedly underestimated' (Das-Munshi et al., 2008, p. 176).

But we also need to be clear that the mixed anxiety and depression label in the Das-Munshi et al. paper was not a diagnosis. It was a sub-syndromal condition that was immediately disqualified once a patient had symptoms of sufficient severity of either anxiety or depression to qualify for one of these disorders. So here we had a 'non-diagnosis' of sufficient severity to create major problems in living that was wiped out once one of the thresholds of formal diagnosis was reached, when a single anxiety or depressive diagnosis took over.

The paper by Das-Munshi et al. (2008) has been well cited (over 100 times) but its subject matter remains isolated in research. It is difficult to understand why there has been so much resistance to defining a mixed anxiety depressive syndrome despite all the evidence of the last 50 years. The question has to be asked: 'If a very common combination of symptoms creates so much pathology in the population at a sub-syndromal level, why is it not recognised at a syndromal one?'

Looking at the way it is dealt with in the psychiatric literature reminds me of the reluctance people now have about referring to the British Isles. There is a tremendous degree of affinity between England, Scotland, Wales, and Ireland but for reasons that are primarily political we do not use 'British Isles' very often. It is felt to be a colonial expression, a hangover from the time of Irish oppression. The people from the island of Ireland are even denoted separately in ethnic population studies; 'the Irish' are a separate group. It is the same with anxiety and depression. We keep them separate because it seems politically correct to do so; depression is a mood disorder; anxiety is a conurbation of like states all associated with high levels of arousal (Craske & Stein, 2016) and so differs from typical depression. So many like to keep them apart, and when those annoying epidemiologists keep reminding us that they are joined together, we just wish they would go away.

In a separate study, Lewis (1991) compared the level of agreement between anxiety and depressive symptoms using a well-known scale (Hospital Anxiety and Depression Scale: HADS) and the Clinical Judgement Scales of the CIS-R. The correlations between anxiety and depression scores in the HADS were 0.59 but only 0.29 in the Clinical Judgment Scales. It could be argued that the psychiatrists were better assessors of anxiety and depression than the patients but in a separate study (described in the same paper) Lewis also found that when psychiatrists (all Maudsley trainees) rated their own anxiety and depression they showed a similar poor correlation. It was therefore reasonable to conclude that psychiatrists were showing bias in finding a degree of separation between anxiety and depression that simply wasn't there.

Lewis therefore concluded from these findings that 'the use of neuroses as, in part, a unitary concept, may be useful and is certainly a legitimate way of describing the current empirical data' (1991, p. 272). Jay Das-Munshi (personal communication) has also suggested that the tendency in insurance-based national systems (e.g., USA, Germany) to bill individually for anxiety and depressive disorders also exaggerates the separation. You could say, if you so wished, that these studies constituted one up for the general neurotic syndrome early in the history of this concept.

1.4   Gavin Andrews and the General Neurotic Syndrome

The general neurotic syndrome suddenly achieved a measure of respectability, if a limited one, by a publication by Gavin Andrews and colleagues in 1990. In this paper, they generously acknowledged and referenced my 1985 publication but Gavin admitted to me (in 2012, when I visited his amazing home close to Botany Bay) that he did not mention that the essential three words in the title were in my 1985 paper. This really did not matter but it was generous of him to confess.

His data came from a study of 15,000 twins involved in the Australian National Health and Medical Research Council Twin Registry, who were also interested in participating in medical research. (It is a pity there was not a UK equivalent as my brother and I would have been keen to be involved). In Andrew's study of 892 twins, and a separate clinic sample of another 165 twins attending for treatment of panic and agoraphobia, there was no evidence of diagnostic stability over time, or to use the words of the authors, no suggestion of 'patterns of co-occurrence of diagnoses being associated with particular syndromes' (Andrews et al., 1990, p. 6). Of more seeming relevance was the background presence of personality vulnerability, so the author had captured the essential parts of the 1985 paper. He took the personality factor one stage further in a later paper:

> In all three domains of information, a general vulnerability factor, associated with personality trait measures of high trait anxiety and poor coping, emerges as a principal cause of these symptoms or disorders, and accounts for the majority of the variation in the comorbidity of symptoms or disorders. This vulnerability factor is shown to be under substantial genetic control. (Andrews, 1996)

He also offered prospects for treatment.

> As these vulnerability factors can be measured, treatment programmes for anxiety and depressive disorders should ensure that they are reduced if relapse is to be inhibited. Prevention programmes, aimed at people with high levels of this personality vulnerability which increases their risk of developing anxiety and depressive disorders, would appear to be practical.

So we, on opposite sides of the globe, had come to the same conclusion. All that remained was for others to follow this up. It was noted in further studies (e.g., Duggan et al., 1996) as a research finding but never appreciated at the clinical level until just recently. Now, after realising that treating resistant depression and anxiety with more and more of the same, it looks at last as though the penny is beginning to drop and the focus will change to examining the personality component (Berk et al., 2018).

1.5 Developments and Changes in Classification since 2010

In the last 15 years, the notion of independent specific psychiatric disorders has received quite a beating. The debates about endogenous and neurotic depression (Kiloh et al., 1972) have all disappeared, and there is increasing knowledge and acceptance of the dimensional nature of psychiatric disturbance. We also have studies that show poor reliability of anxiety and depressive diagnoses as currently described (Andrews et al., 2010) and a host of pharmacological studies that show the terms antidepressants and anxiolytics are inappropriate and 'drugs for depression' and 'drugs for anxiety' are now preferred (Haddad & Nutt, 2020). So why is there such a reluctance to talk about mixed anxiety and depression?

I suggest two reasons. The first is that there has been a gradual separation of anxiety and depression research groups in the last 30 years. The anxiety research groups never study depression and vice versa so there is an innate tendency for each to ignore the other. The second reason is related to treatment. Officially, diagnosis should be made independently of treatment. In the case of anxiety and depression there has been a growing trend for all practitioners to believe that anxiety disorders should be treated by behavioural means and depressive ones by pharmacological ones. So psychiatrists who treat mixed anxiety and depression make the diagnosis a depressive one when they prescribe drugs and an anxiety one when they prescribe cognitive and behavioural methods of treatment. There has also been the influence of training that could be called the Lewis Prediction after his 1991 paper – expressed as 'when symptoms of anxiety and depression are both present the psychiatrist is trained to separate them even when they are of equal importance'.

In this mess of contradiction, the admission that we are mistaken in separating these conditions is almost an admission of failure. The fear that most people might diagnose mixed anxiety and depression and use their discretion as to what treatments they offer is too much to bear. It implies that we know much less about mood disturbance that we think we do.

At the risk of getting too tied up in minutiae these points are worth expanding in the context of the latest classifications.

1.6 Identification of the Co-occurrence of Anxiety and Depressive Symptoms

There has continued to be dispute over the relationship between these symptoms ever since, with only a very slight shift towards the acknowledgement of mixed symptoms as a useful concept. The *International Classification of Diseases* ICD-10 and ICD-11 (world classifications) have allowed mixed anxiety and depressive disorder to be used as a diagnosis but at a very low level when other anxiety and depressive disorders have been excluded. This is the wording in ICD-11:

> Mixed depressive and anxiety disorder is characterised by symptoms of both anxiety and depression more days than not for a period of two weeks or more. Depressive symptoms include depressed mood or markedly diminished interest or pleasure in activities. There are multiple anxiety symptoms, which may include feeling nervous, anxious, or on edge, not being able to control worrying thoughts, fear that something awful will happen, having trouble relaxing, muscle tension, or sympathetic autonomic symptoms. *Neither set of symptoms, considered separately, is sufficiently severe, numerous, or persistent to justify a diagnosis of another depressive disorder or an anxiety or fear-related disorder* (my italics). The symptoms result in significant distress or significant impairment in personal, family, social, educational, occupational or other important areas of functioning. There is no history of manic or mixed episodes, which would indicate the presence of a bipolar disorder. (World Health Organisation, 2018)

The clinician has many other diagnostic options that are considered more acceptable. Dysthymic disorder, a chronic depressive condition, is described clearly in ICD-11 (and essentially the same in DSM-5):

> Dysthymic disorder is characterised by a persistent depressive mood (i.e., lasting 2 years or more), for most of the day, for more days than not. In children and adolescents depressed mood can manifest as pervasive irritability. The depressed mood is accompanied by additional symptoms such as markedly diminished interest or pleasure in activities, reduced concentration and attention or indecisiveness, low self-worth or excessive or inappropriate guilt, hopelessness about the future, disturbed sleep or increased sleep, diminished or increased appetite, or low energy or fatigue. During the first 2 years of the disorder, there has never been a 2-week period during which the number and duration of symptoms were sufficient to meet the diagnostic requirements for a Depressive Episode. There is no history of Manic, Mixed, or Hypomanic Episodes. (World Health Organisation, 2018)

What is most odd about this description is that anxiety symptoms are not mentioned at all – yet another example of the Lewis Prediction that airbrushes every diagnostic conjunction of anxiety and depression away.

If there is a gap in the presence of depressive episodes but there are still many of them, the diagnosis becomes 'recurrent depressive disorder' in ICD-11:

> Recurrent depressive disorder is characterised by a history or at least two depressive episodes separated by at least several months without significant mood disturbance.

A depressive episode is characterised by a period of almost daily depressed mood or diminished interest in activities lasting at least two weeks accompanied by other symptoms such as difficulty concentrating, feelings of worthlessness or excessive or inappropriate guilt, hopelessness, recurrent thoughts of death or suicide, changes in appetite or sleep, psychomotor agitation or retardation, and reduced energy or fatigue. There have never been any prior manic, hypomanic, or mixed episodes, which would indicate the presence of a Bipolar disorder. (World Health Organisation, 2018)

But again there is no mention of anxiety in any form in recurrent depressive disorder, so it will not surprise anyone to read that the descriptions of anxiety disorders do not include even a smidgeon of depressive symptomatology. Generalised anxiety disorder is 'characterised by marked symptoms of anxiety that persist for at least several months, for more days than not', but are 'not a manifestation of another health condition' (presumably including depression), and panic disorder is described by more serious symptoms of anxiety, 'palpitations or increased heart rate, sweating, trembling, shortness of breath, chest pain, dizziness or lightheaded-ness, chills, hot flushes, and fear of imminent death', but again excludes any other health conditions. Similarly, social anxiety disorder is 'characterised by marked and excessive fear or anxiety that consistently occurs in one or more social situations such as social interactions', again with no mention of any depressive components.

1.7 Categories and Dimensions

In trying to set the criteria for the diagnosis of the general neurotic syndrome, I need to emphasise that I am not pretending that this is a very clear category. Almost all psychiatric disorders are best seen as a spectrum from totally absent to strongly present – a continuum with points of diagnosis along the way. The points we choose are ones that are useful to clinicians, not ones that are clear and unambiguous. Bob Kendell emphasised this point many times during his career. Diagnoses are not set in stone, especially in psychiatry; they are merely functional abbreviations that help communication and decision-making (Kendell, 1975a; Kendell & Jablensky, 2003). The diagnosis of the general neurotic syndrome has no status or usefulness unless it helps practitioners to treat their patients. The last chapter of this book explains how this is possible.

It is useful to take an example from medicine to illustrate this, not least as medical diagnoses are often held up as real conditions, as opposed to the fanciful ones of psychiatrists. In the late 1950s, there was a vigorous debate about the status of hypertension in medicine. On the one hand there was Robert Platt, a scion of clinical excellence, who argued that severe hypertension was a genetically determined disease that was completely separate from other conditions in which there was high blood pressure. On the opposite side was George Pickering, an epidemiologist as well as a clinician, who argued that hypertension was a continuously distributed physiological trait, with some people having blood pressure at the upper end of the scale and others further down, but with no clear distinction between the two. It was therefore inappropriate to refer to two groups of people as having either 'normal blood pressure' or hypertension. At the time, there was gladiatorial combat in the *Lancet* between the two antagonists (Platt, 1959; Oldham et al., 1960; Pickering, 1960), all carried out with the utmost politeness, and most commentators, including the editorial staff of the journal (Lancet, 1959), supported the Platt argument.

We now know that Pickering was right and Platt was wrong. There is no genetic basis to hypertension and no clear dividing line between the different hypertension diagnoses, but clinicians, understandably, still find it useful to use higher blood pressures as markers of severity. Even these have come under criticism as it is only night-time recorded (preferably during sleep) hypertension that predicts future cardiovascular events (ABC-H Investigators, 2014).

The hypothesis stated here is that the general neurotic syndrome is similar to hypertension. It represents the extreme of a range and whether it is regarded as clinically useful or a recondite reminder of the past depends on how useful it is in practice. Of course, as all psychiatrists know to their cost, when talking with medical colleagues, we do not have an independent measure of the syndrome like blood pressure to decide what level is pathological, but we do have other assessments that are reliable and sound.

DSM-III and the Generation of New Diagnoses

2

At the time of the instigation of the Nottingham Study of Neurotic Disorder, the revolution instigated by DSM-III was in full swing. 'Neurotic disorders' still received some attention but usually as a precursor to newer (superior) descriptions. Philip Snaith (1991) was still able to entitle the second edition of his book, *Clinical Neurosis*, and explained why in his first chapter.

> The retention of the term neurosis in the title of this book does not imply affiliation to any particular theory or view of the nature of the disorders. On the contrary, it is my purpose to attempt to unite disparate views which have surrounded the concept and to consider how all have contributed to present knowledge although doctrinaire theory has had a retarding effect on progress. (Snaith, 1991, p.1)

He then continued with separate chapters on anxiety, depressive, professional, somatoform, and dissociative conditions, and eating disorders, ending with a chapter on depersonalisation, irritability, and fatigue. His intention was to bring the subject into the framework of the then-developing ICD-10 classification of mental disorders.

2.1 More Personal Experience

In the late 1970s, when I was working in Southampton as a senior lecturer with clinical responsibility for a catchment area to the west of the city, most of the new patients I saw had, in the words of the time, 'neurotic disorders'. The catchment area was relatively affluent and there were many more patients with severe mental illness in hospital then there are today. What struck me most about the patients I was seeing was the commonality between them. I remember time after time writing to general practitioners after a first assessment that the patient had 'a mixed neurotic disorder in which anxious, depressed and phobic symptoms were all present at different times'. Other patients, usually ones presenting for the first time, had symptoms that were much purer in nature. In these instances, I was able to write more confidently that there was a depressive, anxiety, or phobic syndrome with little overlap. With this experience I found the general rubric of the word 'neurotic' to be helpful.

At this time, I was also carrying out clinical research into personality disorder using a new instrument, the Personality Assessment Schedule. (This will be mentioned in more detail later in the book; it plays an important part.) In testing out this schedule, it became increasingly apparent that the group of patients that I classified as neurotic also had significant personality disturbance. So there appeared to be a clear distinction between these groups, summarised in Table 2.1.

Table 2.1 Differentiation of patients in my personal practice between 1975 and 1981

Neurotic group	Non-neurotic group
Had previous episodes from adolescence onwards	Usually presented for the first time. Previous episodes rare
Presented with mixed symptoms (depression, anxiety, phobias, hypochondriasis, panic)	Had clear-cut symptoms of either depression or anxiety, or less commonly, panic and phobias
Had personality disturbance mainly in terms of dependence, obsessionality, and anxiousness	Demonstrated no personality disturbance
Did not respond well to most treatments	Responded well to both drug and psychological treatments
Were difficult to discharge as rarely was there resolution of symptoms. Often re-referred when discharged	Discharged when well, did not re-attend

It was while I was working in Southampton that we organised a randomised controlled trial of the treatment of neurotic disorder (anxiety, depressive, and phobic symptoms) by comparing the clinical outcome and social functioning in patients randomised to day hospital and outpatient care. Day hospitals were promoted strongly for the care of neurotic disabilities as it was felt that the psychologically orientated approach and consequent milieu therapy would be of particular value in day hospital settings. But the results of the study (89 patients) showed no differences between the two approaches (Tyrer & Remington, 1979).

But in looking at the results of the studies, the same findings that I observed in clinical practice were being shown again. Half the patients did well and improved irrespective of setting and the other half continued with symptoms, and this seemed to be related to personality status (although in this study these were not measured). What was abundantly clear was that the inclusion of all anxiety, depressive, and similar symptoms into a general category of neurotic disorder was far from satisfactory.

Before the DSM was published in 1980, there were several indications of what it might contain. David Goldberg, then professor of psychiatry in Manchester, visited Southampton to give a lecture and described the splitting of diagnoses of neurotic disorder that was likely to come after Robert Spitzer had finished his gargantuan task of reforming all psychiatric diagnoses. David, in his inimitable style, pointed out the ludicrous timelines of each diagnosis. We had the separation of panic disorder, which could be diagnosed within a week if you had several panic attacks, from that of dysthymic disorder, which required symptoms of depression to have been present for most of the last two years. In between we had a diagnosis of major depressive episode which required two weeks of suffering before it could be diagnosed, and generalised anxiety disorder, when symptoms had to be present for the last month (also see Figure 1.2). The time limits for phobic disorders did not appear to be so important. David Goldberg presented these proposals in graphical form and in multi-dimensional space; this made them sound even more fantastical than they probably were. But it did not make sense; I did not want to have a clock behind me making the diagnosis (even though it still happens in DSM-5 and ICD-11).

All this work had been generated in the United States and had been triggered by the research of Donald Klein who claimed to have demonstrated 'pharmacological dissection' in showing that imipramine was apparently selective in reducing panic attacks but had no effect on generalised anxiety (Klein, 1964). (He told an impressive story at international meetings: 'The nurses came up to me. "The patients aren't coming to the nursing station any more." I said, "why not?" "They've all lost their panic attacks; is it something you've given them?"'). Yes, of course, imipramine had worked its miracle.

Now we realise that response to antidepressants does not a diagnosis make. The drug words 'anxiolytic' and 'antidepressant' are becoming part of history and have been abandoned in the latest authoritative book on the subject (Haddad & Nutt, 2020). But in the 1970s we were still in the white heat of the psychopharmacological revolution and these new developments were applauded with gusto.

So here was I at this point, as a relatively junior psychiatrist, trying to make sense of a profession in which diagnosis was felt to be an important badge of knowledge. Psychiatrists were esteemed as the decision makers in the mental professional system. Their knowledge of nosology, the science of classification, gave them status and, more importantly, led to (allegedly) correct treatment being given and followed by the rest of the clinical team. Yet here we had earnest discussions at journal clubs in the academic unit at that time disputing diagnosis, especially over the separation of anxiety and depression, not least as, noted in the previous chapter, Sir Martin Roth and his colleagues in Newcastle had published a series of papers claiming a breakthrough in understanding of affective disorders (Gurney et al., 1972; Kerr et al., 1972).

What also bothered me was the relative uselessness of these particular labels when seeing patients in the clinic and writing to fellow doctors with my findings. I also had similar puzzlement when patients were referred to my clinic by psychiatrists and general practitioners and finding that the diagnosis was of very little value unless the writer had disclosed something about the background and circumstances of the patient, with even the occasional mention of a personality profile.

I would not claim to be in any way special in these doubts. Many other psychiatrists, when placed in the same position, have decided that diagnosis in this area of medicine was pretty pointless and abandoned it all together. Dr Ronald Sandison, the original UK enthusiast for psychedelic interventions, was one of these. He was a psychotherapist in Southampton at that time and could not understand my concerns: 'If I don't understand a diagnosis, or feel it is so vague it can apply to anybody how can I treat people successfully?' I asked him. 'That is immaterial', he replied loftily. 'We are in the growth and development business, not the treatment one.'

Of course, that was not going to satisfy me, and these discussions set in mind a great deal of further questions. If this amorphous construction called neurosis, which seemed to be the most common condition in psychiatry, could be harnessed into some sort of order, would we then be able to be more confident about prescribing for, and managing, patients and would we be able to predict their futures?

2.2 Clap of Thunder: The Introduction of DSM-III

Then the skies were opened and down came DSM-III. Would this be the answer to my doubts and questions? It is useful to get DSM-III into context. For younger psychiatrists, it may seem odd that an upgrade of a slightly curious system of classification developed in the

United States that was quite independent of the official ICD (International Classification of Diseases) published by the World Health Organisation, had such an impact when it was published (American Psychiatric Association, 1980).

The reason was psychiatric classification was in a total mess before DSM-III. This was highlighted by what has become known as the Rosenhan experiment. David Rosenhan was a professor of both law and psychology and was particularly concerned about the ethics of involuntary detention. After listening to a lecture by Ronnie Laing, he became interested in testing the ability of psychiatrists to detect severe mental illness even when it was simulated. He conceived the study in two parts.

The first part involved the use of healthy associates or 'pseudopatients'. Rosenhan was one of nine people who took part in this experiment. The others were three psychologists, a psychology graduate student in his 20s, a pediatrician, a psychiatrist, a painter, and a housewife. Three pseudopatients were women, five were men. All of them employed pseudonyms. To make the experiment generalisable, 12 hospitals on the East and West coasts of the United States were chosen: 11 state hospitals and one university one. (It would have been interesting to see if the findings would have differed in any way in hospitals in the central states of the USA).

All the pseudopatients were trained in the same way. They were not specifically asked to imitate the common symptoms of severe mental disorder, only to hint at them. These were Rosenhan's (published) words:

After calling the hospital for an appointment, the pseudopatient arrived at the admissions office complaining that he had been hearing voices. Asked what the voices said, he (or she) replied that they were often unclear, but as far as he could tell they said "empty," "hollow," and "thud." The voices were unfamiliar and were of the same sex as the pseudopatient. The choice of these symptoms was occasioned by their apparent similarity to existential symptoms. Such symptoms are alleged to arise from painful concerns about the perceived meaninglessness of one's life. It is as if the hallucinating person were saying, "My life is empty and hollow." The choice of these symptoms was also determined by the absence of a single report of existential psychoses in the literature. (Rosenhan 1973, p. 252)

In other words, they should have led to some doubt in the psychiatrist's mind that these were in any way typical of psychosis, because clearly, they were not.

Nevertheless, all the 'pseudopatients' were admitted to the hospital for investigation. Each of them was asked to behave normally if they were admitted. They were surprised at the ready acceptance of their curious symptoms. In fact,

none of the pseudopatients really believed that they would be admitted so easily. Indeed, their shared fear was that they would be immediately exposed as frauds and greatly embarrassed. Moreover, many of them had never visited a psychiatric ward; even those who had, nevertheless had some genuine fears about what might happen to them. Their nervousness, then, was quite appropriate to the novelty of the hospital setting, and it abated rapidly. (Rosenhan 1973, p. 253)

So we had a curious situation where patients with fictitious symptoms were admitted readily and then behaved quite normally. But they were not encouraged to leave.

The pseudopatient, very much as a true psychiatric patient, entered a hospital with no foreknowledge of when he would be discharged. Each was told that he would have to get out by his own devices, essentially by convincing the staff that he was sane. The psychological stresses associated with hospitalisation were considerable, and all but one of the pseudo-patients desired to be discharged almost immediately after being admitted. They were, therefore, motivated not only to behave sanely, but to be paragons of cooperation. That their behavior was in no way disruptive is confirmed by nursing reports, which have been obtained on most of the patients. These reports uniformly indicate that the patients were "friendly," "cooperative," and "exhibited no abnormal indications." (Rosenhan 1973, p. 253)

As a condition of their release, all the patients were forced to admit to having a mental illness and had to agree to take antipsychotic medication. The average time that the patients spent in the hospital was 19 days. All but one were diagnosed with schizophrenia 'in remission' before their release. What alarmed Rosenhan was that the label of schizophrenia was affixed to each pseudopatient on very limited assessment, if indeed it can be called an assessment at all. As he put it in his paper 'the evidence is strong that, once labeled schizophrenic, the pseudopatient was stuck with that label. If the pseudopatient was to be discharged, he must naturally be 'in remission'; but he was not sane, nor, in the institution's view, had he ever been sane.'

The second part of his study involved a hospital administration challenging Rosenhan to send pseudopatients to its facility, whose staff asserted that they would be able to detect the pseudopatients. Rosenhan agreed, and in the following weeks, 41 out of 193 new patients were identified as potential pseudopatients, with 19 of these considered suspicious by at least one psychiatrist and one other staff member. Rosenhan sent no pseudopatients to the hospital.

Rosenhan titled his paper 'on being sane in insane places'. It is not a great scientific paper and has been criticised heavily for its many errors and misperceptions (Lilienfeld et al., 2009), but it is described here in detail because I think it did have a big impact on the development of DSM-III. If Rosenhan had carried out his study in the United Kingdom the results may have been very different. The diagnosis of schizophrenia was made much more conservatively there than in the United States, and an important set of data from the UK/US Diagnostic Study a few years earlier (Kendell et al., 1971) had already established the excessive use of the diagnosis of schizophrenia in the Unites States for a wide range of conditions which others just found odd or unusual.

So the stage was prepared for major diagnostic reform and Robert (Bob) Spitzer was there to fill the role of leader. He took over as Chair of the DSM-III task force after frustration in taking part in the anaemic DSM-II classification, introduced in 1968 and still largely dominated by psychodynamic thinking (Spitzer and Wilson, 1968). The DSM-II group was handicapped by many psychiatrists wanting to make their own personal diagnoses based on their clinical judgement, so contained clauses such as 'in the case of diagnostic categories about which there is current controversy concerning the disorder's nature or cause, the Committee has attempted to select terms which it thought would least bind the judgment of the user'. Expressed somewhat differently; 'we have made things as vague as possible so you can easily fit your own pet ideas into the diagnosis'.

Burnished by these experiences, Spitzer took a different approach with DSM-III. First of all, he realised it was important for everyone to have their say, so they did, but he did not necessarily take notice of what they said. Then he organised the meetings in such a way that at the end, before people could leave, Bob got them to agree to a statement of what they had decided.

Alex Spiegel describes this process beautifully:

> Members of the various committees would regularly meet and attempt to come up with more specific and comprehensive descriptions of mental disorders. David Shaffer, a British psychiatrist who worked on the *DSM-III* and the *DSM-III-R*, told me that the sessions were often chaotic. 'There would be these meetings of the so-called experts or advisers, and people would be standing and sitting and moving around,' he said. 'People would talk on top of each other. But Bob would be too busy typing notes to chair the meeting in an orderly way.' One participant said that the haphazardness of the meetings he attended could be 'disquieting'. He went on, 'Suddenly, these things would happen and there didn't seem to be much basis for it except that someone just decided all of a sudden to run with it. (Spiegel, 2005)

Allen Frances, who was also a member of the DSM-III Task Force, describes this similarly in his flowing obituary of Bob Spitzer, except that he exposed the design behind the chaos:

> When Bob began work on DSM III in the mid-1970s, precious little scientific evidence was available to guide how the different disorders should be defined. So Bob created working groups on the various disorders and invited the experts to numerous meetings that all followed the same pattern. He would let us rant and rave in the mornings, blowing off steam promoting competing concepts. Bob would type at blazing speed and was like a magician who seemed to pull DSM III out of a hat—or rather, his computer.
>
> A giant deli lunch would eventually arrive that made everyone drowsy and less argumentative. Bob would then present a beautifully-worded criteria set that captured the best of the morning's suggestions and pacified most disagreements. Thus, DSM III was born. (Frances, 2016, p. 110)

Spitzer kept everyone in the loop afterwards and ensured that agreement to these decisions was maintained until publication. Nevertheless, this was not achieved without a struggle between the Titans of psychoanalytic and conventional psychiatrists. Otto Kernberg led the charge: 'It is a straitjacket and a powerful weapon in the hands of people whose ideas are very clear, very publicly known, and the guns are pointed at us.' (Kernberg, quoted in Bayer & Spitzer, 1985, p.190). But an uneasy harmony was achieved, partly by making personality disorder a separate axis of classification (Axis II) which allowed psychoanalysts much more freedom.

> For the DSM-III task force, and most of American psychiatry, neurosis was an aetiological rather than a descriptive concept. It assumed, as DSM-II noted, an underlying process of intrapsychic conflict resulting in symptom formation that served unconsciously to control anxiety. However, there was no empirical basis for assuming the universal presence of such conflict in those disorders that had traditionally been termed neurotic. There was, for example, no justification for asserting that intrapsychic conflict was always present in what had been denominated 'neurotic depression.' Furthermore, since intrapsychic conflict was present in both those with and those without psychiatric disorders, it could not possibly serve as the basis for discrete class formation, the very purpose of a diagnostic manual. Finally, the task force held that the term neurosis had lost even its earlier specificity as contemporary psychoanalytic theory had shifted its focus of interest from the 'symptom neuroses' to the 'character neuroses (personality disorders)'(Bayer & Spitzer, 1985).

2.3 Hypotheses in the Nottingham Study

The concern I had in 1982, when the ideas behind the Nottingham Study were generated, was that if, as seemed likely, the splitting of many different strands of old neurosis was going to proceed apace, there would be little interest in a different view, namely that the unitary lumping of neurosis still had merit, particularly if it was subsequently found to have a common pathology. I was also singularly unimpressed by the argument that different specific treatments could be selected for each of these new entities. I also needed to have personality assessment at the core of the study if the relationship between neurotic personality and neurotic symptomatology was to be teased out.

2.4 Summary

The theoretical arguments for the acceptance of the general neurotic syndrome have been presented in this chapter, with various lines of independent evidence in support. It is probably one of many Galenic diagnoses that will become increasingly recognised in coming years. But these lofty words alone are not sufficient. Evidence is needed to test out the hypotheses put forward, especially the importance of cothymia and the nature of the personality links. The remaining chapters of this book attempt to provide this evidence in a detailed assessment of the Nottingham Study of Neurotic Disorder.

The Hypotheses
of the Nottingham Study
# of Neurotic Disorder

The reasons for the generation of the Nottingham Study of Neurotic Disorder were at their core a series of important questions:

(1) Is personality an important component of what has been called 'neurosis'?

(2) Is it clinically useful to regard mixed anxiety and depression (which from henceforth in this book is called cothymia) as a syndromal rather than a sub-syndromal condition?

(3) Is there evidence that the anxiety and depressive symptoms in neurosis differ in their response to different treatments?

(4) Do patients with neurosis and personality difficulties get better over time or do their problems persist?

These questions would answer the issue of whether there was value in maintaining the neurotic concept, formulated as described earlier as the general neurotic syndrome.

To answer the first of these questions, it was necessary to record personality status reliably; to answer the second, cothymia needed to be diagnosed as a clinical syndrome; to answer the third, it was necessary to carry out a randomised controlled trial of treatments; and to answer the fourth, a long period of follow-up was needed.

3.1 Reliable Assessment of Personality Disorder

In 1982 there were no world-wide accepted measures of personality disorder. Many assessment interviews had been created, including Bernreuter's Personality Inventory (Bernreuter, 1931), the Rorschach Inkblot Test (Rorschach, 1921), the Minnesota Multiphasic Personality Inventory (Hathaway & McKinley, 1940), the Thematic Apperception Test (Murray, 1943), and the 16PF Personality Questionairre (Cattell & Stice, 1957). But none of these was focused on personality disorder and there were many doubts about their value in a personality-disordered population.

In any case, DSM-III had just been published and it was clear that this revolution in diagnosis would lead to new measures, especially for personality disorder. I wrote to Bob Spitzer at the New York Psychiatric Institute and he was interested and attentive, admitting that he was in the process of developing an instrument for recording personality disorder and asking for advice. It was subsequently published and, in its later version with Michael First as the first author, became the most widely used instrument in the 1990s (First et al., 1995).

But we were keen on getting the Nottingham Study started and there was also concern that any instrument linked to the DSM classification would be likely to change over time. We needed a measure that was reliable, comprehensive, and unchanging for the duration of a follow-up study. I had developed a measure a few years earlier called the Personality

Assessment Schedule (PAS) which seemed to satisfy these requirements (Tyrer & Alexander, 1979; Tyrer et al., 1979). This instrument is not particularly well known, partly because it has not been made available commercially or through an academic institution, but also because in the course of its development I realised that training in its use was very important before it could be scored properly. I therefore wanted tight control of training before the instrument could be more widely used. (This is not a very sensible way of popularising a scale as the wider the use the better, but I have stuck to it over the years, and those who want to use it have to be determined.)

The Nottingham Study was envisaged in 1981 and initiated in 1982, but did not begin recruiting patients until later in 1983. This was not a study carried out in a high-powered academic centre with many resources, and the hypotheses could have been considered as reactionary rather than progressive, so getting the resources and people to support it was not easy. At the time, I was working as a consultant psychiatrist in Nottingham and had recently transferred my extra-hospital activities to general practice. This was professionally the most satisfying time of my career in respect of patient care (Tyrer, 2013) and I need a section to explain why and also describe the advantages that the clinics held for the Nottingham Study.

There were two big advantages of the PAS. It was not tied to any other system of recording personality so could not be changed or suddenly made redundant by a successor, and the conclusion of the analysis of the data suggested that personality could be placed on a single spectrum, as the results 'supported the concept of personality disorders as being at the extreme of a multidimensional continuum' (Tyrer & Alexander, 1979, p. 166). Thus, the PAS was equipped to record personality disturbance in terms of severity as well as type, and this was to be of particular value for the future of the Nottingham Study.

3.2 The Importance of Recording Cothymia

As cothymia is defined as the simultaneous presence of anxiety and depressive symptoms, it was necessary to include patients in the study who had both anxiety and depressive diagnoses. Good diagnosis could readily be achieved by using the most reliable diagnostic system at the time, DSM-III, and formally scoring anxiety and depression using the Structured Clinical Interview for DSM-III that had just been introduced (Spitzer & Williams, 1983).

But the DSM-III did not make any allowance for comorbidity, so mixed anxiety and depression in any form was not permitted. Instead, a hierarchy was created in which panic disorder trumped dysthymic disorder and both panic and dysthymic disorder trumped generalised anxiety disorder. Of course, this was anathema to the thinking of the Nottingham Study and as we had recorded both anxiety and depressive disorders at baseline assessment, we were able to include cothymia as an additional diagnosis.

3.3 Testing Whether Anxiety and Depressive Symptoms Differ in Their Response to Treatment

This hypothesis could only be tested adequately in a randomised controlled trial. Such trials are not easy to set up and need large numbers to yield definitive results. As we were trying to test efficacy in both anxiety and depression separately and together (cothymia) we needed to test three groups. As specific efficacy had been claimed for antidepressants in the treatment of panic disorder it was necessary to have patients with panic disorder included in the study also. Psychological treatments were also to be included if the trial was to be a comprehensive one.

3.4 Long-Term Outcome

Long-term outcome studies in mental health are difficult. It is very different with physical health disorders, when patients often feel privileged to be involved in doctors' concern for their care. It is even better when you have doctors themselves involved in the research, as they tend to be even more assiduous in agreeing and providing data for follow-up studies.

In October 1951, Richard Doll and Austin Bradford Hill sent a questionnaire on smoking habits to all registered British doctors. In the previous year, they had just demonstrated the association between smoking and carcinoma of the bronchus and wanted to know more about the effects of smoking long-term. They sent out 59,600 questionnaires: 41,024 replies were received and 40,701 (34,494 males and 6,207 females) provided enough data to be included in the follow-up (Doll & Bradford Hill, 1954). You would never get figures like this in a psychiatric follow-up study. Short follow-up was followed by further questionnaires about changes in smoking habits up to 2001. The study has yielded a mass of information, not the least of which is that even if smokers reduce or stop their cigarette consumption late in life, it still makes them less likely to get bronchial carcinoma than if they persist (Doll et al., 1994).

I met with Richard Doll in 1982 when he was visiting Nottingham; he was a friend of my father and had stayed with us in the past. I talked to him about the Nottingham Study and three pieces of advice he gave were followed in the study. Firstly, he emphasised the need to have simple measures of outcome. 'Its easy for me, because most of my studies involve death as an outcome, and that is unequivocal. But you can't do this in psychiatry. But you can choose a simple outcome that everyone can recognise. Are people after treatment ill or no longer ill? Choose a simple measure of illness.'

Secondly, he emphasised the need for a placebo control in the randomised trial, and, thirdly, he pointed out the advantages of long-term follow-up. 'If a treatment only gets people better for a few weeks and they get worse afterwards there is not much point in choosing it. And if you don't know the natural history of a condition you will be tripped up time and time again in making premature conclusions.'

3.5 How to Recruit Patients to the Study?

Most patients with common mental disorders are treated entirely in primary care. If a hospital or outpatient population is chosen, it may not be representative. This is one of the criticisms that could be directed against the Newcastle Group studies of anxiety and depression; they were carried out with inpatients. I wanted to avoid studying a population that could be criticised as being at the severe end of the spectrum of mood disorders.

Fortunately, a suitable population was available in Nottingham and a service was available to treat them. Nottingham, unlike many other areas in the country in the nineteenth century, was not allowed to place its mental hospital somewhere in the back of beyond. The 'out of sight, out of mind' mentality was there but could not be followed through on as the city was compelled to build its hospital services within the city boundaries, so had to choose local, not distant. In the end it was decided the new hospital would be built on the top of a hill at the northern limit of the town at a place called Mapperley (ever since called Mapperley Top). It was not an ideal site, 'long and narrow, bordered by a main road to the east and a deep valley to the west' (Mindham, 2020). It might have been a nightmare to create but fortunately it had a highly competent architect in the form of George Hine to design it. The 'long corridor' hospital subsequently had a celebrated 114-year history, helped greatly near its end by the pioneering community work of Duncan MacMillan, a dour but far-seeing Scot, who was one of the first twentieth-century psychiatrists to recognise that autonomy is good for patients and seclusion from the world is not.

But because the hospital was local, it attracted considerable stigma. When patients were admitted they were often taken there in one of a fleet of cream-coloured vans linked to the hospital. This was noted immediately by Nottingham mothers; children's bad behaviour was often controlled with a threat to arrange 'a visit from the yellow van' (Tyrer, 2008a). So the hospital, despite its mainly good reputation among the profession, became a place to avoid, and this unfortunately extended to its fellow hospital, St Ann's, built in 1934, and its outpatient clinics close by. People generally did not like going there for appointments and the setting was glum.

However, it was very different in the 1980s in general practice. Spanking new premises were being opened up every year. They were closer to people's homes and very pleasant to visit. Several consultants and I set up, with agreement and great enthusiasm from GPs, psychiatric clinics in general practice settings. These were both refreshing and efficient. I got to know the GPs well and we had frequent conversations about patients at crucial times in their care – so much better than a stilted letter (Darling & Tyrer, 1990). From the point of view of the Nottingham Study, these clinics were ideal as patients were referred there earlier in the course of their problems and so I was in a better position to assess the general problems of neurosis before too many other labels had been applied.

This form of care was possible in the 1980s as resources were adequate and there was still considerable enthusiasm for developing new forms of community care. At this time, I was holding 19 clinics a month across Nottingham and the yellow bags (the ones provided by the hospital and containing the notes for each clinic – no extra technology then) clearly replaced the yellow vans. The service was effective and efficient and before long most of my colleagues had joined in. We subsequently had strong evidence that this enterprise reduced the demand for inpatient beds (Tyrer, Turner & Johnson, 1989; Williams & Balestrieri, 1989), even though they created some extra referrals (Jackson et al., 1993; Tyrer, Ferguson & Wadsworth, 1990). During one special period in 1987, admittedly only for two days, I had no patients in hospital; everyone was an outpatient. But these were the days when the community cycle was in top gear and running downhill. It has been an uphill struggle ever since and though for a short time the Department of Health was interested in moving forward with general practice clinics across the country, it was only in Scotland where this was considered seriously as an alternative provision. Despite this, in other countries, the idea of these clinics in primary care or in separate non-psychiatric settings is still being developed (Carr & Donovan, 1992; Grenyer et al., 2018; Anjara et al., 2019). The key is to have senior people in these settings who have extensive knowledge of the patient (Darling & Tyrer, 1990); just placing a single mental health practitioner in the clinic is not sufficient (Emmanuel et al., 2002).

Seeing patients in general practice clinics was ideal for the Nottingham Study, as referrals often took place much earlier than in normal outpatient practice. From the beginning of the planning of the study it was decided only to include patients who were not taking any treatment at the time of assessment. This reduced the pool of potential participants but made the cohort a more homogeneous one.

3.6 Generating the Randomised Controlled Trial and Follow-Up

The trial plan that I developed was a complex one and needs justification. I was aiming to examine the general concept of neurosis with a particular emphasis on anxiety and depression. Even if my hypothesis was correct and combined anxiety and depression was found to be a very different condition from the individual diagnoses of these conditions, if there was an obvious diagnostic difference in response to treatment (as Klein, 1964, 1981, and others would argue), then this would justify the existing diagnostic system. This made it necessary to include antidepressant and antianxiety treatments, preferably drug and psychological, and because the design of the study was unusual there had to be a placebo arm in the randomised treatments. (Having support from Richard Doll here was very valuable when dealing with the local ethics committee, which initially refused to contemplate a placebo component until I emphasised that Richard deemed it essential.)

The selection of diagnoses was also important. The most difficult was the choice of the right diagnosis of depression. The umbrella diagnosis of 'major depressive episode' was felt to be too vague and would overlap with more serious depressive disorders, so instead the diagnosis of dysthymic disorder was chosen, and as its alternative title was given as 'depressive neurosis' in DSM-III (American Psychiatric Association, 1980, p. 220), it was felt to be a more appropriate diagnosis to include.

As noted in all classifications of depression, there was no mention of anxiety symptoms in the DSM-III description (American Psychiatric Association, 1980, p. 221) but all practitioners recognised that anxiety was a component to the diagnosis. This was subsequently summarised very neatly by Gene Paykel:

> In the last 20 years dysthymia has proved a useful concept, delineating a form of mood disorder which can produce many problems and have an adverse impact on the life of the sufferer, and it has generated much research. There is a high rate of comorbidity, particularly of anxiety disorders and substance abuse. The majority of dysthymics ultimately also develop an episode of major depression, and such episodes, so-called double depression, have a worse prognosis than pure major depression, both in respect of remission and of recurrence. There appears therefore to be continuity between dysthymia and major depression. The *DSM-IV* definition rules out an episode of major depression in the first 2 years, but the *ICD-10* definition does not. In practice the differentiation of dysthymia from milder chronic major depression or from the residual symptoms with partial remission which frequently occur after major depression, is difficult and may be artificial. (Paykel, 2008)

There was also the problem of the sample size. Three diagnoses and five treatments were eventually chosen, but when calculations were made and it was decided to only recruit 210 patients, an obvious criticism was made that this might lead to a Type II error (i.e., a true difference that was not identified as the sample size was too small). In the end, we decided to have a constrained randomised sample in which a computer-generated algorithm allocated the 210 patients in the following fashion (Table 3.1).

Table 3.1 Randomised trial and treatment numbers

Treatment Number
Diazepam 28
Dothiepin 28
Placebo 28
Cognitive and behaviour therapy 84
Self-help 42
TOTAL 210

It will immediately be noticed that the numbers in the drug groups are small. This was because the intention at the beginning of the trial was to continue it as a follow-up study after 10 weeks. The self-help and psychological treatments were clearly known to the investigators but double-blind methodology meant that the drug groups could not be identified. After 10 weeks, if people felt they had responded to their allocated treatment, they were encouraged to continue it 'in the same mode'. This translated into the 84 allocated to drug therapy continuing drug treatment in the form of dothiepin (without breaking the blind of the original allocation), 84 continuing with CBT or similar psychological treatments, and 42 continuing with self-help. (Dothiepin was chosen as at that time it was the most commonly prescribed antidepressant in the UK; Boots Pure Drug Company also provided the placebo and diazepam capsules of identical appearance.)

3.7 Duration of Treatment

At the time when we carried out the Nottingham Study, it was commonplace to have the end-point of a trial when the last treatment was given. We anticipated later concerns about adverse effects, partly because of evidence we had found that withdrawal symptoms with diazepam could be identified when withdrawing after only six weeks of treatment (Murphy, Owen & Tyrer, 1984). So we set the duration of treatment of all types to be six weeks only, and then to gradually withdraw medication (and CBT) so that at 10 weeks all patients were on no therapy.

3.8 Inclusion and Exclusion Criteria

There is always a battle, when deciding on whom to recruit to a trial, between those who would like a completely representative population with as few exclusions as possible, and those who would prefer a tightly selected homogeneous group who represent the best population to test your hypotheses. We decided to err in favour of the former in the Nottingham Study.

We only had the following exclusion criteria:

(i) existing diagnosis of major depressive episode after the Structured Clinical Interview for DSM-III (SCID) assessment,

(ii) patient taking psychotropic drugs at time of assessment,

(iii) past history of schizophrenia or manic-depressive psychosis.

3.9 Assessments in the Randomised Trial

Because the Nottingham Study required assessments of both anxiety and depression, as well as a detailed interview about personality status, it was decided at the outset that all assessments should be carried out by face-to-face interviews. This sounds straightforward but it is not, and nowadays digital technology is increasingly being used in place of direct contact. This is a pity, as the clinical interview, even a research clinical interview, yields so much more than a set of ratings on a scoresheet. Particularly in a follow-up study, frequent contact with the same investigator often leads to an easy informal relationship that promotes excellent understanding. Indeed, at later assessments, when we asked each patient what had helped them most over the course of treatment, several identified our researchers as top of their list, even though no treatment of any sort had been provided by them.

At baseline in the randomised trial, six assessments were made. The procedure in each case was a two-stage process. The first stage involved screening the patient for eligibility at assessment at the general practice clinic by a consultant (me) or a senior registrar. If the patient was regarded as eligible and was willing to take part in the trial, the Structured Interview for DSM-III was given and assessments made for all depressive and anxiety diagnoses. If the patient satisfied the requirements for the diagnosis of panic, dysthymic or generalised anxiety disorder, or any combination of these, the next sealed envelope was opened and one of five treatments disclosed, the three drug treatments (A, B or C), cognitive behaviour therapy (CBT), or self-help. The second interview, carried out within a day or so of the first, involved a visit from a previously trained research assistant (all junior psychiatrists), who administered the Personality Assessment Schedule and five other scales:

1 The Comprehensive Psychopathological Rating Scale (CPRS) (Åsberg et al., 1978).

(Although I like to avoid acronyms, because this scale has a long title I will abbreviate this to CPRS in most of the references that follow). This is a 65-item observer-rated scale that includes both the assessment of symptoms (40 items) and observed behaviour (25 items) with each item scored on a four-point scale. It has the advantage of being truly comprehensive, being able to assess present psychiatric state, the severity of a full range of symptoms, and the change in symptoms over time. It was said to take about 50 minutes to administer but when being used frequently this time could be shortened greatly. It also has a summary four-point rating (CPRS-Global). Greater severity is shown by higher scores.

Although most of the scales selected for the Nottingham Study have been continued to be used to the present day, the CPRS is the only one that has fallen out of favour.

2 Montgomery and Åsberg Depression Rating Scale (MADRS)

If the CPRS is the also-ran in the rating scale stakes, the MADRS is the Olympic champion (Montgomery and Åsberg, 1979). It was derived directly from the CPRS, but the poor chap at the back of the field never gets much credit. The MADRS scale has been cited nearly 10,000 times in the scientific literature and is the most highly cited paper ever published in the *British Journal of Psychiatry*. It records 10 items from the CPRS and has expanded the scoring to make change easier to detect so there is a maximum score of 6 for each item. Later studies suggest scores of 7 to 19 indicate mild depression, 20–34 moderate depression and >34 severe depression (Herrmann et al., 1998).

3 The Brief Anxiety Scale (BAS)

This scale was developed by me and tested out with other colleagues in studies carried out in the early 1980s (Tyrer, Owen & Cicchetti, 1984). It is the anxiety equivalent of the MADRS as it also contains 10 items from the CPRS and scores them in a similar fashion with a maximum score of 6 for each item. Two of the items (inner tension and reduced sleep) are the same as in the MADRS, and yet again this illustrates the overlap between anxiety and depression described in earlier chapters. The scale correlates well with self-ratings of anxiety (and depression), as does the MADRS (Evenden et al., 1996), but the agreement is not quite strong enough to regard a self-rated measure as redundant (0.76–0.83).

4 Hospital Anxiety and Depression Scale (HADS)

This scale was only introduced in 1983 (Zigmond & Snaith, 1983) but has been cited over 25,000 times in the scientific literature. It is a simple 14-point scale that has 7 anxiety and 7 depression items.

Assessing depression and anxiety with two rating scales for each might be thought unnecessary but here the Lewis Prediction also applied. Any tendency of the assessing psychiatrists to overstate anxiety when present with depression would be counteracted by the self-rating HADS scales.

5 Personality Assessment Schedule (PAS)

The Personality Assessment Schedule is listed as the Appendix of this book. It is a 24-item scale that has not been used widely. This is partly my fault. As noted earlier in this chapter, when testing the schedule we noted that reliable assessment of personality with the scale was highly dependent on training. Those very new to personality assessment tended to overscore on some items and minimise others. There was also the problem of the nature of the informant (for example, if this was the recently estranged spouse of a person the assessment of the other might contain elements of bias). In general, we found women to be better than men in making assessments (Brothwell, Casey & Tyrer, 1992).

Because of these concerns, the PAS was only released for formal studies after negotiation and only a handful of studies outside our group have used it, with perhaps the most interesting being the study by Manuel Cuesta and colleagues (2002) that suggested that the schizoid (detached) dimension in the PAS in patients with first-episode psychosis was associated with the development of negative symptoms in schizophrenia. The PAS studies have included comparisons with other instruments and these in general have supported its structure and likely accuracy, especially with regard to its slightly shorter version, the Quick Personality Assessment Questionnaire (Hill et al., 2000; Germans, Guus & Hodiamont, 2011, 2012).

The other advantage of the PAS was that it did not change over time. If other instruments had been used, they would have had to be updated with DSM-III-R and DSM-IV replacements. Because the PAS recorded severity of personality disorder as one of its regular components, it was also very much in tune with the new ICD-11 classification of personality disorder (Tyrer et al., 2019), and a separate validation study was carried out to allow the baseline PAS scores to be converted into ICD-11 severity categories (Tyrer et al., 2014). This has allowed ICD-11 categories to be incorporated into the results.

3.10 Setting Up the Financial Aspects of the Trial

One of the main problems in carrying out research that is not a natural development from pre-existing studies is that funding is difficult to obtain. This was particularly difficult in my position at the time as I was an NHS consultant, not with an academic title, although I had general encouragement to carry out research. What follows in this section might be useful advice for others placed in the same position.

First, you need some independent advice that what you are planning is not completely inappropriate or simply not feasible. If you persist at this point you will only achieve the epithet of being stupidly pig-headed and stubborn and the work will go nowhere. (Some people said that to me anyway, but because I had good opposing voices I could continue). I spoke to several colleagues, principally Gene Paykel, at that time Professor of Psychiatry at the University of Cambridge, and he was supportive. Bob Kendell in Edinburgh was similar in his encouragement. 'Why not go ahead', Gene said, 'but you will find it a struggle to get the money.' I decided not to go for the major grant funders on the grounds that they would turn the application down in view of my status at the time, and as the world was then so attuned to the splitting of so many diagnoses one that was unashamedly linked to 'the lumpers' would get short shrift.

So, a range of different options were considered for funding, the details of which are summarised at the end of this book. But it was not only the funding that mattered. Far more important were the people who supported the project from the beginning, many of them junior doctors in training posts, who carried out extra work in learning the assessment procedures, training on the Personality Assessment Schedule, visiting patients at home repeatedly over the period of follow-up, and generally providing encouragement when problems arose.

Accumulating the necessary funds for a large trial is analogous to moving to a new house and finding out that a piece of wasteland at the back of the house is masquerading as your garden. You go outside, plant a spade in the rock-hard ground, get stung by nettles, pricked by thistles, and coiled in bindweed and feel like giving up. But if you plan, a little at a time, things begin to change. Better still, once you have made some progress, others notice, give suggestions and maybe even some help, and before long the waste area looks a little like a proper garden. At this tipping point everyone realises that the garden is a real creation, offers plants and more suggestions, and finally you have something of beauty to see when you look out of your bedroom window.

Once we had sufficient funds to start the trial, and received a positive ethical opinion, we were able to start. The first patient was recruited to the study in October 1983. We did not have an 'end day' for recruitment as we needed to continue until all 210 patients were randomised, and this was not until August 1987.

Chapter 4

Interpretation of the Results of the 1988 Lancet Randomised Trial

The results of the 10-week randomised trial were published in the *Lancet* in July 1988 (Tyrer, Seivewright, Murphy et al., 1988). The main findings at this point did not include any analysis of the general neurotic syndrome as this was not a term that would have been understood by the average reader and would have just led to confusion. The results were presented in a standard manner, focusing on the effects of the five treatments (Figure 4.1) and of the outcome of the three diagnostic groups (Figure 4.2).

The summary of the trial's findings was expressed thus:

> There were no important differences in treatment response between the diagnostic groups, but diazepam was less effective than dothiepin, cognitive and behavioural therapy, or self-help, these treatments being of similar efficacy. Significantly more patients in the placebo group took additional psychotropic drugs in the 10 week period, and those allocated to dothiepin and cognitive behaviour therapy took the least. (Tyrer, Seivewright, Murphy et al., 1988, p. 235)

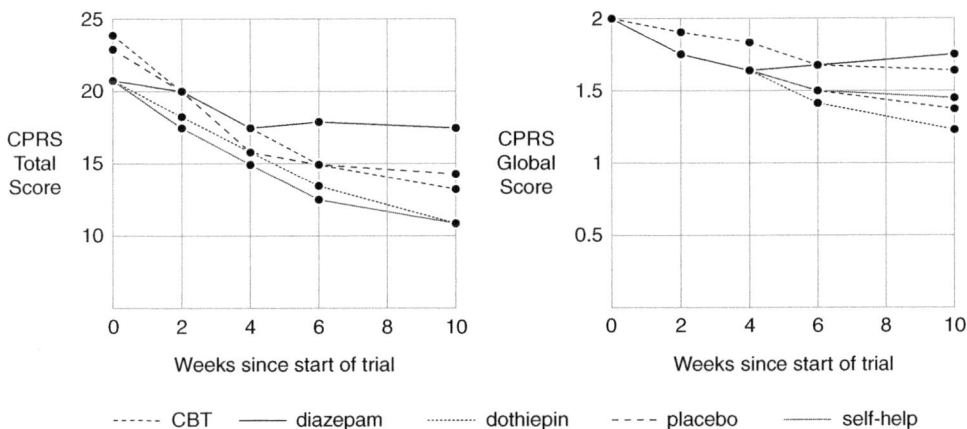

Figure 4.1 Results of the Nottingham Study of Neurotic Disorder Trial separated by randomised group for each of the main outcomes (adapted from Tyrer, Seivewright, Murphy et al., 1988a with kind permission of the *Lancet*)

NB. Significant differences in diazepam-treated patients in CPRS total scores (F = 2.91; df 4,196; P = 0.023), CPRS global score (F = 2.7; df 4,177; P = 0.03) and MADRS scores (F = 2.47; df 4,196; P = 0.046)

Patients allocated to placebo were more likely to take additional treatments (31%) in the trial than the other groups, diazepam (15%), dothiepin (7%), CBT (9%), and self-help (18%) (odds ratio 3.4, 95% CI 1.2–9.8) (X^2 = 7.1; df 1, P < 0.01)

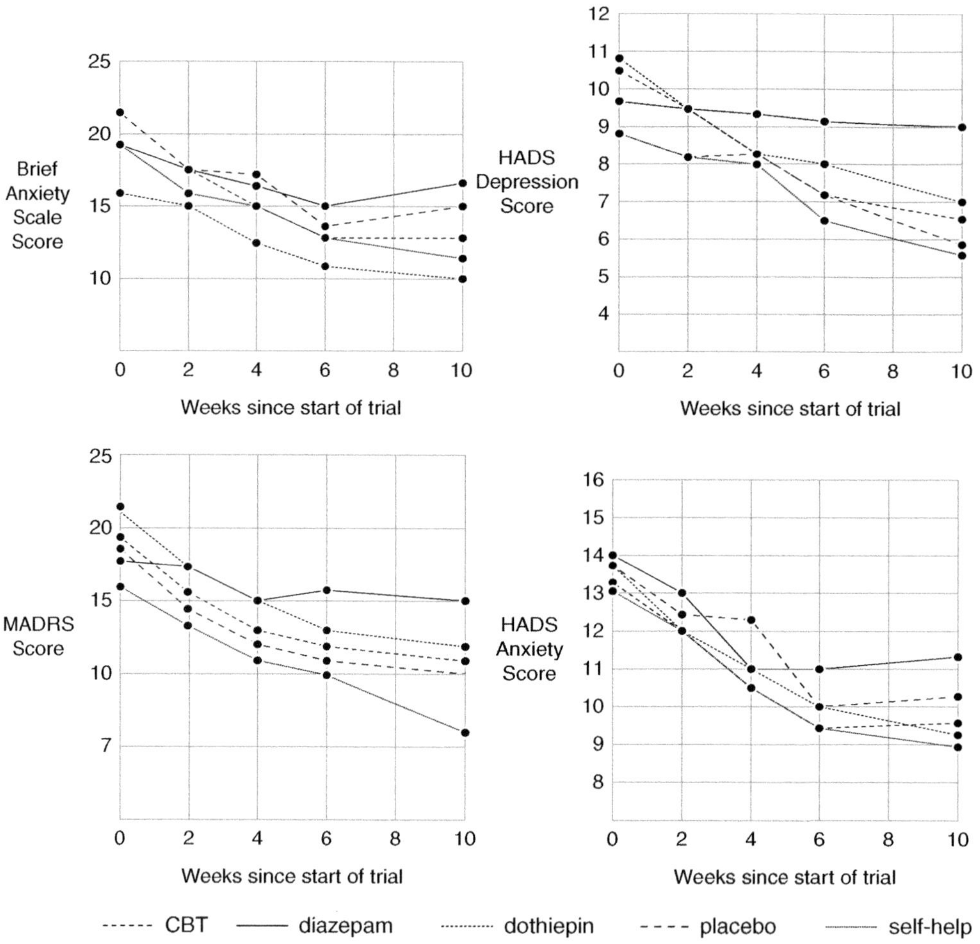

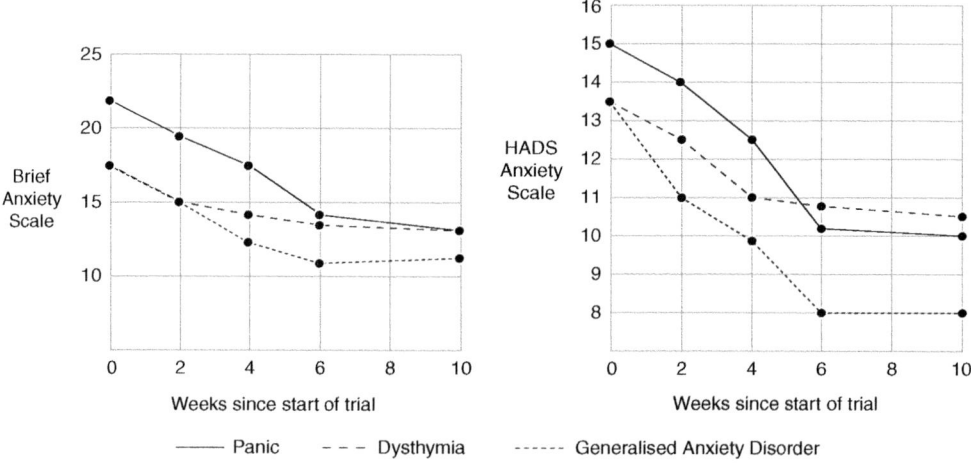

Figure 4.1 (cont.)

Figure 4.2 Results of the Nottingham Study of Neurotic Disorder randomised trial separated by initial DSM diagnosis (adapted from Tyrer, Seivewright, Murphy et al., 1988 with kind permission of the *Lancet*)
NB. Mean CPRS scores were lower in patients with GAD (14.1, 95% confidence interval 12.4–16.0) than in dysthymic disorder (18.1, 95% CI 16.1–20.3) and panic disorder (17.4, 95% CI 15.5–19.3) (F = 4.6; df = 2,198; P = 0.012)

4.1 Baseline Data in Randomised Trial

Table 4.1 Baseline data in all treatment groups in randomised trial

No. of patients	Diazepam 28	Dothiepin 28	Placebo 28	CBT 84	Self-help 42	Total 210
Gender	M 8: F 20	M 9: F 19	M 6: F 22	M 34: F 50	M 8: F 34	M 65: F 145
Age (median)	33	36	32	36	35	35
Social class 1–2	2	5	6	13	2	28
Social class 3	9	4	7	17	8	45
Social class 4	11	12	6	32	16	77
Social class 5	6	7	9	22	16	60
Main DSM diagnosis						
Dysthymia	10	11	8	23	13	65
GAD	11	10	10	28	12	71
Panic disorder	7	7	10	33	17	74
Mean CPRS score	20	19	24	21	20	21
Mean MADRS score	18	22	19	19	16	18
Mean BAS score	20	18	22	20	19	19
Mean HADS-A score	15	15	15	14	13	14
Mean HADS-D score	8	14	9	11	9	10

4.2 Differences in Diagnosis

Table 4.2 Adjustment of diagnosis after accounting for cothymia

Initial	Dysthymic disorder	Generalised anxiety disorder (GAD)	Panic disorder	Cothymia
Main diagnosis at randomisation (n)	65	71	74	–
Revised diagnosis after adjustment for comorbidity (n)	9	70	60	71
Change	−56	−1*	−14	+71

* One patient with GAD had a virtually equal depression diagnosis so counted as cothymia.

4.3   Distribution of GNS Positive Cases by DSM-III Personality Status

Table 4.3 Personality status of patients with GNS at baseline

DSM-III PD diagnosis	% of total assessed (n=181)	% of those with GNS	Significance of GNS vs non-GNS numbers (x^2)
Histrionic	12.7	15.2	ns
Paranoid	12.2	12.1	ns
Dependent	10.5	22.2	$P < 0.001$
Avoidant	10.5	19.7	$P < 0.01$
Antisocial	9.4	4.5	ns
Borderline	9.4	6.1	ns
Obsessive-compulsive	8.8	16.7	$P < 0.02$
Passive-aggressive	6.6	6.1	ns
Narcissistic	6.1	4.5	ns
Schizotypal	4.4	4.5	ns

Note: each patient can have more than one personality disorder.

Personality status was recorded with the Personality Assessment Schedule (PAS) at baseline. This was completed by assessors who were unaware of GNS status or initial diagnosis. The PAS also includes an algorithm to convert the personality status, if all information is available, into the DSM-III personality disorder diagnoses. The results were not unexpected. Those with DSM-III diagnoses of dependent, avoidant, and obsessive-compulsive disorders were more likely to have the general neurotic syndrome (Table 4.3).

4.4   Clinical Outcomes

The graphical presentation of the results best explains the differences between the three DSM diagnoses and the outcomes of each of the five treatments. The only significant result was that patients on diazepam had poorer outcomes than all other groups. We are sure that this is because we included the period of withdrawal as well as that of active treatment so that any symptomatic benefits were partly erased during withdrawal.

But it is important to stress that the numbers in the study were still relatively small and so only big differences were likely to be significant. We also were hiding the main reasons for the differences in outcome between the diagnoses. What is clear from the scores on the two anxiety measures, the Brief Anxiety Scale and the Hospital Anxiety and Depression Scale – Anxiety Section (4.2), is that panic disorder has more severe symptoms than generalised anxiety disorder. A score of between 16 and 17 on the Brief Anxiety Scale indicates pathological anxiety (Tyrer et al., 1984) and one of 8 or more is commonly accepted as the threshold for pathological anxiety (Stern, 2014), and the mean scores in the Nottingham Study were well above these thresholds. Still, the patients with panic disorder had scores nearly 50 per cent higher than those with generalised anxiety disorder. Those with dysthymic disorder, allegedly a depressive disorder but one we have already noted to consist mainly of cothymia, had baseline levels similar to those with generalised anxiety but improved less well over the 10-week period than the other two groups (Figure 4.1), so explaining their overall higher ratings.

4.5 Differences in Treatments

As the summary of the paper and Figure 4.1 indicate, no differences were found between the treatments in the randomised trial apart from an inferior result with diazepam. So why did diazepam do so badly compared with the other treatments? The answer is simple, although it has taken many years for most people to under-stand why. Diazepam, ever since it came to be regarded as an addictive drug even in therapeutic dosage, has been recommended to be taken for four weeks and then gradually reduced. That is what we did in the Nottingham Study, unlike most other studies in which improvement is measured while patients are taking the drug. But we now know that withdrawal symptoms can occur after stopping benzo-diazepines after only a few weeks (Murphy et al., 1984), and that is precisely what happened in the Nottingham Study. There was improvement on the anxiety measures and total CPRS score at first but when the drugs were gradually withdrawn this improvement disappeared and patients' scores returned to very similar levels to those at baseline.

4.6 Reaction to Publication

There was a generally positive reaction to the *Lancet* publication, but some predictable criticism from Donald Klein in New York. He had four major complaints: (1) the numbers in the study, particularly the ones taking drug treatments, were too low so a Type II error was very likely; (2) the drug doses of dothiepin and diazepam were trivial; (3) he objected to the statements that 'panic disorder was a quantitatively more severe form of generalised anxiety disorder rather than a specific entity' and that dothiepin was a 'typical antidepressant'; and (4) he concluded that 'the study produced an expensive Type II error with no useful therapeutic or nosological implications' (Klein, 1988).

We responded by pointing out that, as the dosage regime was a flexible one starting with a low dose, the dosage at six weeks was the better one to record; there was evidence of gradual improvement over the six-week period; dothiepin was indeed a tricyclic antidepres-sant (the most commonly used in the UK at the time); and there was absolutely no suggestion of specific treatment/diagnosis differences over time with any of the measures recorded. If there was a Type II error, there should have been at least an inkling of a difference shown in some of the depression and anxiety scores; there was none (Tyrer, Seivewright, Ferguson et al., 1988).

But Klein was right in pointing out that the numbers of patients with panic disorder treated with antidepressants were not large enough to reach firm conclusions. Other experts also suggested that dothiepin was not a typical tricyclic antidepressant, but this was a footling comment; dothiepin is directly related to amitriptyline.

Others commented, sometimes with glee, that the trial showed that all treatments for anxiety and depression were useless as placebo was just as good. But placebo was not just as good – its outcome path was similar to diazepam for the CPRS global score and anxiety scores (Figure 4.1) and those in this group took significantly more additional treatments than the others (Tyrer, Seivewright, Murphy et al., 1988).

But the important result, hidden from the publication in the *Lancet*, was that the general neurotic syndrome, showing strong overlap with dysthymic disorder, had a worse outcome than other diagnoses. In other words, cothymia, the diagnosis that everyone chooses to ignore, was much more resistant to short-term treatment. Dysthymic disorder, despite having no mention of anxiety in its definition, was riddled with anxiety. Almost all the patients at baseline with this condition had generalised anxiety as well, but our other hypotheses were concerned with more acceptable diagnostic conditions and so in our published work we felt it best to stay with the conventional labels. But throughout we still recorded the progress of those with the GNS.

The study also showed that personality disorder had little impact on the outcome measures. Those with more severe personality disorders had higher symptom scores on all measures both at baseline and 10 weeks but the improvement was similar in all groups (Tyrer, Seivewright, Ferguson et al., 1990). This is, in itself, an important finding, as subsequent studies have often challenged the now fully accepted view that personality disorder has no influence on the outcome of depression. The doubters and the believers have been reconciled in a definitive paper by Newton-Howes et al., (2014). The key issue is the length of follow-up.

Although the randomised trial finished after 10 weeks, if the patients had made progress and wished to continue in the same mode of treatment they were prescribed antidepressants in the three drug groups, encouraged to stay with psychological treatments in the CBT group, and with self-help and other similar supports in the self-help group. This was not in any way forced, but as the greatest improvement in the whole 30 years was found in the first 10 weeks, it was not surprising that many followed the suggested procedure.

4.7 Placebo Response

Much of the reaction to the *Lancet* publication was related to the placebo response. The nature of the positive elements of the placebo response had not been fully appreciated in 1988, and the hard-nosed reaction was that the trial must be valueless if other treatments were not shown to be superior. But the setting of the trial was very much in keeping with practice at that time. A treatment was prescribed, progress assessed after a few weeks, and if improvement was achieved the treatment was withdrawn. With this design, placebo effects may be more marked.

We now know that much of the improvement in mental symptomatology can be explained by the placebo response. The 30 per cent improvement in symptoms shown in most groups in the trial illustrates a common law of mental health – taking part in a randomised trial is good for you, no matter to what treatment you are allocated.

4.8 Conclusions about the General Neurotic Syndrome after the 10-Week Trial

The general neurotic syndrome in the *Lancet* was the disguised elephant in the room. He was there, if you were clever enough to look for him, but he had already set down a marker if you noticed him or not. Mixed anxiety-depression (cothymia) was a highly important diagnosis that would not be going away in a hurry.

The Medium-Term Outcome of the General Neurotic Syndrome

The main hypothesis of the Nottingham Study was that the general neurotic syndrome would have a more complex and likely poorer outcome in the long-term, so follow-up data were critical in evaluating this. Assessments were made of the main outcome measures at 16, 32, 52 (one year) and 104 weeks (two years) after randomisation. At five years, assessment was only made through examination of the patients' GP and hospital notes.

5.1 Outcome in the Shorter Term

The results of the clinical outcomes are shown in Table 5.1 and Figure 5.1. Whereas those without the GNS improved by over 50 per cent in the year after randomisation, those with the definite syndrome improved by only 25 per cent in the same period, and similar differences were shown at five years. The regression analysis showed the significant difference evident as early as 10 weeks in those with the GNS was not found with other variables, including personality status (Table 5.1) (Tyrer, Seivewright, Ferguson et al., 1990).

Although the treatments in the study were similar after 10 weeks (apart from diazepam), a subsequent analysis of the CBT therapists in the trial showed that the patients treated by the therapists who were judged to be highly competent by the main supervisor (David Kingdon), had significantly better outcomes at two years than the others (Kingdon et al., 1996). At two years, the patients who had improved most were those treated by these competent therapists.

Table 5.1 Summary of regression analysis on outcome in first two years of Nottingham Study

Variable	10 weeks	16 weeks	32 weeks	52 weeks	2 years
N	180	180	178	179	173
Initial CPRS score	0.30 (P < 0.01)	0.36 (P < 0.001)	0.21 (P < 0.04)	0.23 (P < 0.03)	0.38 (P < 0.005)
General neurotic syndrome (Y/N)	0.18 (P < 0.02)	0.27 (P < 0.0005)	0.20 (P < 0.004)	0.16 (P < 0.03)	0.17 (P < 0.02)
Personality disorder (Y/N)	0.05 (NS)	0.04 (NS)	0.07 (NS)	0.00 (NS)	0.14 (P = 0.05)
Initial observed anxiety (BAS)	0.09 (NS)	−0.02 (NS)	0.21 (NS)	0.26 (P < 0.025)	0.01 (NS)

The full analysis can be found in Table 7 of Tyrer et al. (1992).

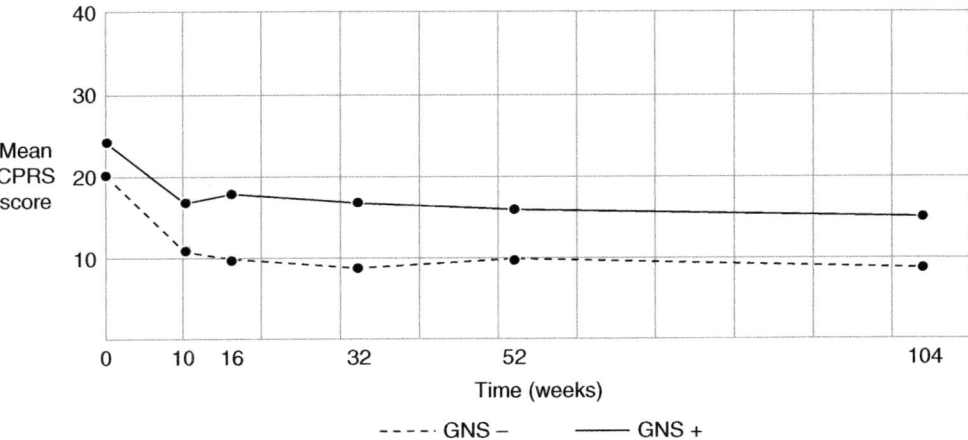

Figure 5.1 Mean changes in total psychopathology scores (CPRS) for patients with the general neurotic syndrome (GNS+) (n = 66) and those without (GNS–) (n = 115). The GNS positive cases represent scores of ≥ 6 on the GNS scale

5.2 Five-Year Outcome

The 5-year assessment was made, after ethical approval, by examination of medical records by the same investigator who carried out the 12-year assessments, my wife, Helen. (I should here stress that Helen is a stickler for accurate recording and independent working, and made absolutely sure that she knew nothing about the baseline status of the patient when she made her assessments.)

Exactly five years after original referral, she contacted the relevant mental health units and general practice surgeries and, if permission was given, visited to record the details of all treatments received. After all data had been collected on each patient, she made a judgement of overall outcome using a standardised scale (Global Outcome Scale), as will be discussed.

The same data were recorded at 5 years and again at 12 years, including the numbers of contacts with all health professionals for psychiatric disorder over the period, the contacts with the general practitioner for non-psychiatric conditions (as best as could be done from the content of the notes), the number and length of psychiatric admissions and day-hospital attendance, all psychotropic drugs treatment received and the total time the patient was not taking psychotropic drugs during the 5 years (after completing the original trial). Private medical consultations were not recorded but in the Nottingham area these constituted a small proportion of total contacts.

To ensure that the Global Outcome Scale was being consistently and reliably assessed, 10 sets of records were evaluated independently by PT. All were scored similarly.

The results were very similar to other studies of this group of common disorder – about one third do very well, another third improve a little, and the final third remain unwell. This was first reported in an early study by Hans Eysenck (1952).

It was appreciated that examination of records alone was not a substitute for direct contact with the patient, and that the outcomes recorded were primarily those of service receipt. Nevertheless, the results of the later assessments, when both global

Table 5.2 Global outcome in 182 patients after five years

Outcome category	Description of outcome	Number (%)
1. Very good	No psychiatric contact with either general practice or psychiatric services since initial period of care (up to nine months)	50 (27)
2. Good	Some contact for psychiatric problems in general practice or psychiatric clinics but at least half time well	57 (31)
3. Fair	Frequent contact with services for psychiatric problems for more than half of time of follow-up, but intensity of care not great (e.g., short period of daycare, many outpatient contacts but no inpatient care)	38 (21)
4. Poor	Little or no time in follow-up period well. Intermittent contact as outpatient or day-patient	28 (15)
5. Very poor	Continuously ill with frequent contact with all parts of psychiatric services or death from deliberate self-harm	9 (5)

outcome and clinical ratings were recorded, showed a surprising level of agreement between them. We also examined the data at two years and again the service outcome at that time correlated well with the clinical outcome recorded by rating scales (Tyrer et al., 1993).

5.3 Analysis of Data

In this part of the study, we were especially looking at the success of the baseline data in predicting the outcome at five years. The method chosen by our excellent statistician, Tony Johnson of the MRC Biostatistics Unit in Cambridge, was polychotomous stepwise logistic regression. This allows the creation of different models to examine data that are not binary ones, so many ordered outcomes can also be included. Thus we were able to examine all the baseline variables; age, sex, marital status (married, single, separated or divorced or widowed), social class, randomised treatment group (drug, psychological treatment, and self-help), original DSM-III diagnosis (dysthymic, generalised anxiety, and panic disorder), duration of symptoms, categorisation of original episode as new or recurrence, precipitating factors into four groups (none, loss, conflict, and addition events), personality disorder classified by type and severity using the PAS classification, and the presence or absence of the general neurotic syndrome (GNS).

5.4 Results

The results of the regression analysis showed two major findings; (i) older age and the identification of a recurrent disorder at baseline led to an odds ratio of 4.20 for a poor outcome, and (ii) the combination of a personality disorder and the GNS had a similar odds ratio of 3.28 for a poor outcome. An interesting subsidiary finding was that higher scores on the main clinical outcome at 10 weeks, the Comprehensive Psychopathological Rating Scale (CPRS) also predicted a poor outcome (odds ratio 2.88) (Seivewright et al., 1998).

It is worth reflecting on these findings. They show that a good global outcome was achieved in those who had a new episode of anxiety or depression, who were young, and who improved greatly in the original randomised controlled trial (when they may have received a placebo). This is exactly what you would expect in the sometimes misunderstood diagnosis, adjustment disorder, defined as 'a condition that arises in response to a stressful event or situation', and 'which resolves spontaneously when the stressor is removed or when a new level of adaptation is reached' (Casey, 2018, p. 2).

But all the patients in the Nottingham Study had a formal DSM-III diagnosis of panic or dysthymic or generalised anxiety disorder, which are above adjustment disorder in a hierarchical system of classification. The conclusion must be that at least a proportion of the patients seen would have been best classified as adjustment disorders rather than the more serious conditions. As one might have expected, those with the general neurotic syndrome were more likely to have had recurrent episodes and so fit in with the other data.

5.5 Contacts with services in first five years in GNS patients and those with personality disorder

The service contacts of patients with scores of four or more on the GNS scale are shown in Table 5.3, and those separated by initial ICD-11 personality disorder in Table 5.4. Those with possible or definite syndrome had significantly more GP and outpatient appointments than those without the syndrome and also had longer periods of day care and more contacts with community nurses. The only significant difference in the other group was a higher level of contact with social workers in those with personality disorders, although the trends were generally similar in both GNS and personality disordered patients.

5.6 Diagnosis at Baseline and Service Outcomes

Cothymia was also examined in the five-year data and, as this was postulated to be central to the GNS, the service data for this group were needed (Table 5.5).

The results gave some support to the expectation that cothymia would lead to more service contacts but they were not striking (Table 5.5). Appointments for non-psychiatric illness in primary care and non-psychiatric admissions were more frequent in cothymic and dysthymic patients. There were also more psychiatric admissions and contact with social workers.

5.7 Summary of Findings at Five Years

We concluded at the time we published most of these findings that the pithy description of Surtees and Barkley (1994) that the outcome in these disorders was 'future imperfect' was an

Table 5.3 Service outcomes separated by general neurotic syndrome (GNS) status five years after randomisation

Follow-up time point Service contacts		GNS <4	GNS 4–5	GNS ≥6	P[a] difference	P (linearity)
0–5 years						
		N: Mean ± SD	N: Mean ± SD	N: Mean ± SD		
No. of GP/OP appts for psych illness		94: 14.0 ± 15.6	30: 18.9 ± 18.0	65: 18.3 ± 16.6	0.031	0.011
No. of GP/OP appts for non-psych illness		94: 22.6 ± 18.2	30: 21.9 ± 20.5	65: 26.7 ± 17.8	0.165	0.111
Length of day care (weeks)		94: 1.34 ± 5.8	30: 5.17 ± 15.0	65: 5.1 ± 12.4	0.009	0.002
Weeks of non-psych hospitalization		94: 0.54 ± 0.96	30: 0.63 ± 1.0	65: 0.71 ± 1.3	0.585	0.302
Weeks of psych hospitalization		94: 0.29 ± 1.4	30: 0.27 ± 1.0	65: 0.17 ± 0.82	0.818	0.541
No. of admission		94: 0.65 ± 1.1	30: 0.90 ± 1.4	65: 0.92 ± 1.3	0.326	0.155
Months free from psychotropic medication		99: 47.0 ± 18.9	31: 46.5 ± 19.5	70: 39.8 ± 21.3	0.194	0.083
		N (%)	N (%)	N (%)		
Contact self-help groups	No	89 (94.7)	27 (90.0)	62 (95.4)	0.579	0.915
	Yes	5 (5.3)	3 (10.0)	3 (4.6)		
Contact social workers	No	84 (89.4)	25 (83.3)	52 (80.0)	0.225	0.099
	Yes	10 (10.6)	5 (16.7)	13 (20.0)		
Contact community psychiatric nurses	No	43 (45.7)	7 (23.3)	17 (26.2)	0.014	0.008
	Yes	51 (54.3)	23 (76.7)	48 (73.8)		
Contact psychologists	No	89 (94.7)	29 (96.7)	61 (93.8)	1.000	0.848
	Yes	5 (5.3)	1 (3.3)	4 (6.2)		

[a] Exact test

Table 5.4 Service outcomes separated by baseline personality disorder

		No PD	PD	P[a]
0–5 years				
		N: Mean ± SD	N: Mean ± SD	
No. of GP/OP appts for psych illness		118: 14.7 ± 13.6	66: 19.5 ± 20.4	0.173
No. of GP/OP appts for non-psych illness		118: 24.4 ± 19.5	66: 20.0 ± 16.5	0.991
Length of day care (weeks)		118: 3.36 ± 10.7	66: 3.30 ± 10.2	0.383
Weeks of non-psych hospitalization		118: 0.39 ± 1.1	66: 0.53 ± 1.1	0.778
Weeks of psych hospitalization		118: 0.62 ± 1.1	66: 0.58 ± 0.9	0.651
No. of admission		118: 0.75 ± 1.2	66: 0.82 ± 1.2	0.699
Months free from psychotropic medication		126: 44.8 ± 20.2	69: 42.6 ± 20.2	0.785
		N (%)	N (%)	
Contact self-help groups	No	109 (92.4)	64 (97.0)	0.176
	Yes	9 (7.6)	2 (3.0)	
Contact social workers	No	109 (91.5)	50 (75.8)	0.007
	Yes	10 (8.5)	16 (24.2)	
Contact community psychiatric nurses	No	40 (33.9)	25 (37.9)	0.631
	Yes	78 (66.1)	41 (62.1)	
Contact psychologists	No	115 (97.5)	60 (90.9)	0.072
	Yes	3 (2.5)	6 (9.1)	

[a] Exact test

accurate one. Forty per cent were still adversely affected through persistent or recurring symptoms. The evidence that older patients presenting with neurotic symptoms had a worse outcome was also consistent with data from Surtees and Barkley's study.

The finding that personality status, linked to the general neurotic syndrome, was an important clinical indicator of longer term outcome was consistent with other evidence (Duggan, Lee & Murray, 1990; Quinton, Gulliver & Rutter, 1995).

The evidence that the general neurotic syndrome linked to a personality disorder diagnosis was a better predictor than personality disorder alone suggests the identification of dependent and obsessional features of personality abnormality (the anxious-fearful cluster C in the DSM classification) and the presence of cothymia and family history of a similar disorder all contribute to poor prognosis.

It was interesting to note that many of the other possible predictors of outcome were negative. The negative predictors are at least as informative as the positive ones. In particular, the initial diagnostic group contributed little of importance to the prediction

Table 5.5 Service outcomes separated by DSM-III diagnosis after adjustment for cothymia

		Dys	GAD	Panic	Cothymia	P[a] (difference)
		N: Mean ± SD	N: Mean ± SD	N: Mean ± SD	N: Mean ± SD	
0–5 years						
No. of GP/OP appts for psych illness		8: 11.4 ± 12.4	68: 15.4 ± 17.4	57: 17.8 ± 15.8	61: 15.6 ± 16.1	0.214
No. of GP/OP appts for non-psych illness		8: 16.4 ± 11.7	68: 24.2 ± 19.5	57: 20.9 ± 17.9	61: 27.9 ± 19.0	0.108
Length of day care (weeks)		8: 0 ± 0	68: 2.44 ± 7.7	57: 4.25 ± 11.5	61: 3.39 ± 12.0	0.460
Weeks of non-psych hospitalization		8: 0.38 ± 0.5	68: 0.84 ± 1.3	57: 0.35 ± 1.0	61: 0.70 ± 1.1	0.048
Weeks of psych hospitalization		8: 0.25 ± 0.7	68: 0.34 ± 1.6	57: 0.12 ± 0.7	61: 0.23 ± 0.9	0.783
No. of psychiatric admissions		8: 0.63 ± 1.1	68: 0.87 ± 1.3	57: 0.44 ± 0.7	61: 1.03 ± 1.4	0.054
Months free of psychotropic medication		8: 51.1 ± 19.5	69: 43.8 ± 21.1	59: 43.3 ± 19.0	68: 45.1 ± 20.7	0.832
		N (%)	N (%)	N (%)	N (%)	
Contact self-help groups	No	8 (100.0)	65 (95.6)	52 (91.2)	58 (95.1)	0.744
	Yes	0 (0.0)	3 (4.4)	5 (8.8)	3 (4.9)	
Contact social workers	No	5 (62.5)	59 (86.8)	53 (93.0)	48 (78.7)	0.037
	Yes	3 (37.5)	9 (13.2)	4 (7.0)	13 (21.3)	
Contact community psychiatric nurses	No	4 (50.0)	27 (39.7)	16 (28.1)	21 (34.4)	0.436
	Yes	4 (50.0)	41 (60.3)	41 (71.9)	40 (65.6)	
Contact with psychologists	No	7 (87.5)	63 (92.6)	56 (98.2)	58 (95.1)	0.286
	Yes	1 (12.5)	5 (7.4)	1 (1.8)	3 (4.9)	

[a] Exact test

of outcome, with only a little added by cothymia. Only 40 of the patients had no precipitating events but this did not lead to a better outcome as might have been expected. The duration of symptoms was also not predictive as might have been expected.

After only five years, it was too early to predict the course of the general neurotic syndrome but these early data suggested that people with this core neurotic condition:

(i)   were high users of primary care services,
(ii) were high users of psychiatric care,
(iii) could be identified better by their core symptoms and personality than by duration and initial manifestation,
(iv) had a fluctuating course.

The evidence that the general neurotic syndrome conferred a better prediction of service outcome than personality disorder diagnosis alone was not entirely unexpected. The elements of personality dysfunction in the GNS – dependence, anxiousness, and obsessionality – are ones that have subsequently been shown to be related to treatment seeking (Tyrer, Mitchard et al., 2003), whereas the others are associated with treatment resistance or indifference.

Overall, the results at five years allowed the following tentative comments to be made on the basis of global outcome and service contacts:

(1) DSM-III diagnosis does not predict outcome.
(2) Personality disorder does predict outcome but the strength of this is reinforced by including the general neurotic syndrome.
(3) Initial improvement in symptoms is associated with a good outcome and suggests a re-diagnosis of adjustment disorder.
(4) Those with the general neurotic syndrome are the highest users of general practice and secondary psychiatric care services.

6 Chapter

The General Neurotic Syndrome at 12 Years

The patients in the Nottingham Study after 12 years had not been assessed in person since the two-year outcome. In planning the assessments at 12 years, additional information was felt to be needed to reinforce the collection of previous data (Table 6.1).

Table 6.1 Measures included in the 12-year follow-up of the Nottingham Study

Data collected at 2 years	Data collected at 12 years	Reasons for 12-year data inclusion
Personality assessment (PAS)	Personality assessment (PAS)	To check on stability of personality disorder[*]
Comprehensive Psychopathological Rating Scale (CPRS)	Main rating outcome measure	Main rating outcome measure
Montgomery and Åsberg Depression Rating Scale (MADRS)	Important secondary outcome	Important secondary outcome
Brief Scale for Anxiety (BAS)	Important secondary outcome	Important secondary outcome
Hospital Anxiety and Depression Scale (HADS-A and HADS-D)	Important secondary outcome	Important secondary outcome
DSM-III diagnosis	Not specifically recorded	Simple dichotomous outcome (Richard Doll choice)
GP contacts	Important service outcome	Important service outcome
Out-patient psychiatric contacts	Important service outcome	Important service outcome
Non-psychiatric GP contacts	Important service outcome	Important service outcome
Hospital admissions	Important service outcome	Important service outcome
Suicide attempts and deaths	Key clinical outcome	Key clinical outcome

Table 6.1 (cont.)

Data collected at 2 years	Data collected at 12 years	Reasons for 12-year data inclusion
Psychological services	Important service outcome	Important service outcome
Social function	Not recorded	New: Recognition that social function is a key measure in neurotic disorder
Global outcome scale	Recorded at 5 years (important service outcome)	Also recorded at 12 years
Neurotic disorder outcome scale (NDOS)	Not recorded	New: A clinical outcome measure
Costs of care	Not recorded	New: Important for public health

*Personality change over the 30 years is not reported here but the results showed personality disorder as a diagnosis was very unstable over time (Yang, Tyrer, Johnson & Tyrer, (2022).

The three additional measures recorded at 12 years were social function, the Neurotic Disorder Outcome Scale, and a full analysis of costs (Table 6.1). Social function was the most significant of these. We included it as at the time there was accumulating evidence that many of the negative consequences of mental illness are tied up with poor social function (Casey et al., 1985; Casey & Tyrer, 1986; Fredman et al., 1988). There are many good measures of social function but most of these are quite long. In the end we chose the Social Functioning Questionnaire (SFQ)(Tyrer et al., 2005).

This could be considered a lazy choice as I was the main author. It may have been, but after considerable discussion over a previous schedule that I had developed with Marina Remington in Southampton (Remington & Tyrer, 1979) (also discussed in some detail with Steve Platt, an international expert on the subject), it was felt to be an appropriate measure as it covered all the essential elements of social function. It was also very short and, as the 12-year follow-up was a long interview, particularly because much of the time was taken up with personality assessment, brevity was a boon. Since the late 1990s, the Work and Social Adjustment Scale (Mundt et al., 2002) has become the most widely used short instrument and this only has five items. Nevertheless, detailed study of the Social Functioning Questionnaire (SFQ) suggests that it, and a shorter form of only five questions, is a very good initial screen for personality disorder (Tyrer, Yang et al., 2021). In itself this is very interesting as it appears that, despite social functioning being influenced by many factors, personality appears to be the major one.

6.1 Cold-Calling

This section of the chapter could be regarded as an aside. It is only concerned with the acquisition of data in follow-up studies, but it is of interest to any investigators involved in any follow-up work. It is now commonplace to ask for written consent when carrying out research studies. This cannot be done in advance even though it would be desirable in follow-up studies. If a patient agrees to have an interview two years after signing a consent form when the time comes for the interview no consent form will be valid and a new one has to be obtained. So, although in the Nottingham Study patients were usually informed about the date of the next assessment and agreed or did not agree to be seen again, it challenged the memory much more when the interval between the face-to-face interviews was 10 years after the last one. The other problem frequently found in long-term follow-up studies is a change of patient's address. The standard way of approaching a patient is to send a letter to the last known address (it may have changed greatly in 10 years, let alone since the 1990s). This gives the opportunity for the patient to agree to a follow-up interview or refuse if preferred.

There are several problems with this from the researcher's point of view. The patient may not receive the letter because they have moved address, they may receive it and have no idea what it is all about and toss it in the bin, or they put it aside and do not reply (even though a stamped addressed envelope was added to the letter). None of these actions constitutes refusal to be seen. Although a second letter was sent if there was no reply to the first, exactly the same responses may be shown.

This is where the vexed issue of cold-calling comes in. What should happen if there is no response of any sort to the standard approaches? This is the procedure we used eventually – exact wording – after discussion with the Nottingham Ethics Committee:

(a) Standard letter written to last known address inviting a follow-up appointment. If the patient chose refusal of contact in their response no further action was taken;

(b) If the patient replied positively within four weeks a follow-up appointment was made;

(c) If no reply or patient thought to have moved the Family Health Service Authority (FHSA) was contacted to determine any change of address;

(d) If no reply, and original address thought to be correct, a second copy of the standard letter was sent with a hand-written letter explaining the project again;

(e) Similar approaches made to new addresses of patient if thought to have moved;

(f) If no response made the patient was either telephoned or called upon without prior appointment to see if patient still living at address and to introduce project. If the patient agreed the follow-up interview took place at this time, and if the patient refused, no further action was taken.

Phase (f) of this procedure is cold-calling, and was only used when no other contact had been established with the patient and all letters (which included stamped addressed envelopes on every occasion) had failed to be returned. (Tyrer, Seivewright, Ferguson et al., 2003, p. 239).

If we had relied on standard guidance in the 12-year follow-up, the study could well have foundered at that point. In Table 6.2, the results of cold-calling are shown. Of all the patients seen, 45.6 per cent were cold-called; our results would have been severely compromised if we had only had a follow-up rate of 54.4 per cent, the completion rate that would have been achieved without cold-calling. Those who needed cold-calling were very similar to those who were seen using normal procedures. Only social class (classes 1 and 2 were responsive to letters) showed any differences (Table 6.2).

Since the 12-year follow-up, the views about cold-calling have become more liberal. The success of a public health research project, that all would normally support, can be compromised by restrictions imposed by well-meaning barriers protecting the absolute

Table 6.2 Comparison between initial and cold-call responders for selected initial variables

Baseline variables	Initial responders (n = 100)	Cold call responders (n = 84) (%)	Summary statistics (95%CL)*	Statistic and P-value**
Gender: Male	29	30 (36)	1.0	$\chi^2 = 0.9$, P = 0.33
Female	71	54 (64)	1.36 (0.73, 2.53)	
Personality disorder				
Present	35	29 (35)	1.0	$\chi^2 = 0.0$, P = 0.97
Absent	62	52 (62)	0.99 (0.53, 1.87)	
NK	3	3 (4)		
Social class				
1	6	1 (1)	} 1.0	
2	13	5 (6)		Ns
3	20	20 (24)	0.32 (0.10, 0.96)	(except for social class 1&2 vs rest)
4	34	33 (39)	0.33 (0.11, 0.92)	$\chi^2 = 4.5$ (after Yates correction), P<0.035
5	27	25 (30)	0.34 (0.11, 0.99)	
Marital status				
Married	42	32 (38)	1.0	$\chi^2 = 1.3$, P = 0.52
Separated/divorced/widowed	29	21 (25)	1.05 (0.51, 2.18)	
Single	29	31 (37)	0.71 (0.36, 1.42)	
Initial treatment				
Drug	45	28 (33)	1.0	$\chi^2 = 3.8$, P = 0.15
CBT	34	40 (48)	0.53 (0.27, 1.02)	
Self–help	21	16 (19)	0.82 (0.36, 1.83)	

Table 6.2 (cont.)

Baseline variables	Initial responders (n = 100)	Cold call responders (n = 84) (%)	Summary statistics (95%CL)*	Statistic and P-value**
Initial diagnosis				
GAD	36	27 (32)	1.0	$\chi^2 = 2.0, P = 0.37$
Dysthymia	25	29 (35)	0.65 (0.31, 1.35)	
Panic	39	28 (33)	1.04 (0.52, 2.11)	
Age at entry				
<20	5	4 (5)		
20–29	28	26 (31)		
30–39	30	29 (35)		
40–49	25	15 (18)		
50–59	8	7 (8)		
60+	4	3 (4)	1.26 (−2.11, 4.63)	$t_{180} = 0.74, P = 0.46$
Mean	35.9	34.6		

*Odds ratios or differences between means, reference categories indicated with OR = 1.0.
**chi-squared for binary and categorical variables, chi-squared for trend for original variables; t-test or Mann–Whitney test for continuous variables
Reproduced from Tyrer, Seivewright, Ferguson et al, (2003) with the permission of BMJ Publishing Group.

right of patients to refuse. All well and good, but if the initial consent form contained words such as 'this study involves long-term follow-up for the following reasons (these are then specified). The success of the study will depend on your agreement to be seen in the future. This will always be done at a time to suit you. Please let me know, at least in principle, if you are prepared to support this arrangement.' This would at least set the markers in advance. And of course, circumstances can change. One of the patients seen at 30 years told me on the doorstep: 'I am sorry. I am dying of cancer and do not feel I can properly answer your questions; I do not think they would help you very much.' We commiserated by his door and reflected on the awfulness of fate and the lottery of life, and then I went on my way. He died five weeks later. Of course, he was right to refuse and his data would not have been helpful, but at least we had some human contact.

The current attitude to cold-calling may be reflected in a quotation from a recent review of the subject:

> although the restriction of cold calling aims to promote patient privacy, given the complexity and collaborative nature of medicine, the individual provider may not have sufficient information or resources to facilitate recruitment decisions. We call for institutions to abandon strict cold call policies, and adopt recruitment strategies that balance patient choice, privacy, and research success. (McHugh, Swamy & Hernandez, 2018, p. 390)

I think the key word here is 'balance'.

6.2 Costs

These are discussed here at the only time in this book, as it was only at 12 years that we had a comprehensive assessment of the costs of the study carried out by Gerhard Knerer as part of a Medical Research Council Collaborative Group investigating complex interventions. We have always lived in times of rationing when it comes to health services. There are always more demands on resources than we can possibly fill. But we should always remember that providing these resources is like filling a watering can with a small leak in the bottom; some resources are wasted and will never be recovered.

In examining the justification for the use of the general neurotic syndrome, the total cost over the 12 year period was the preferred statistic.

The results of the cost analyses show some important findings, some of which are counter-intuitive, and in interpreting these it must be remembered that costs tend to scatter over a wide range and only large differences are found to be significant.

The findings that showed important differences in costs can be summarised as (i) those with dysthymia (original diagnosis) or cothymia (adjusted diagnosis) incur greater costs than others, (ii) patients presenting with a recurrent disorder also create greater costs than those presenting for the first time, and (iii) those with the general neurotic syndrome incur costs more than 50 per cent greater than those without the syndrome.

Perhaps, equally importantly, the severity of symptoms (as measured by scores on each of the scales) does not have an impact on costs, or personality disorder and disturbance. This, although showing the linear tendency for costs to increase with each increment of severity, also does not account for much of the cost differences. In this respect, the clinical outcomes, which are related strongly to initial symptom severity (see Table 6.5), differ from the cost findings.

The results in Table 6.3 show univariate analyses but because many of the variables cross-correlate it is necessary to carry out multivariate analyses also. These are not shown here but the results of the multivariate model showed that three factors – the general neurotic syndrome, initial diagnosis (and cothymia), and the presence of

Table 6.3 Univariate predictors of 12-year costs ($) *The GNS threshold score was set at 4 in this analysis

Variable	n	Total cost ($) per patient	Standard deviation (SD)	Significance of differences
Randomised treatment				
Drug therapy	84	11,517	12,112	
CBT	84	12,669	20,529	0.854 (ns)
Self-help	42	11,308	8,736	
Gender				
Male	65	11,013	12,480	0.565 (ns)
Female	145	12,350	16,732	
Age on entry				
<30 years	70	10,452	13,459	
30–44 years	91	12,104	18,542	0.103 (ns)
45 years or older	49	13,742	11,729	
Social class				
1 & 2	28	8,196	7,412	
3	45	14,295	24,418	0.439 (ns)
4	77	10,999	9,976	
5	60	13,115	15,561	
Marital status				
Married or cohabiting	83	11,888	18,596	
Divorced, separated, widowed	56	12,823	13,038	0.860 (ns)
Single	71	11,293	13,406	
Diagnosis on entry				
Dysthymia	65	15,747	23,110	
Generalised anxiety disorder	71	11,446	11,473	P = 0.037
Panic disorder	74	9,059	8,594	
Type of episode				
New	142	9,368	9,250	P<0.001
Recurrent	68	17,298	22,988	
General neurotic syndrome*				
Absent	106	9,260	9,987	P = 0.011
Present	104	14,663	19,298	

Table 6.3 (cont.)

Variable	n	Total cost ($) per patient	Standard deviation (SD)	Significance of differences
CPRS score on entry				
0–16	52	9,895	10,301	
17–21	59	10,875	13,275	P = 0.56
22–28	50	14,408	23,239	
29	49	12,857	12,614	
MADRS score on entry				
0–15	61	9,919	9,730	
16–19	49	14,758	24,492	P = 0.61
20–25	49	11,835	13,389	
26	51	11,734	11,527	
BAS score on entry				
0–15	55	12,192	12,871	
16–19	55	10,746	14,232	P = 0.62
20–25	53	11,612	11,019	
26	47	13,395	22,831	
HADS-D on entry				
0–8	75	10,207	6,136	
9–12	64	15,172	14,101	P = 0.365
13–15	46	10,018	4,435	
16–22	25	12,368	11,171	
HADS-A on entry				
0–8	25	10,488	8,248	
9–12	43	10,630	11,297	P = 0.354
13–15	66	11,661	11,922	
16–22	76	13,389	21,492	
Personality status on entry				
No personality dysfunction	88	10,537	12,492	
Personality difficulty	52	11,758	11,573	P = 0.20
Simple personality disorder	50	13,829	23,479	
Complex personality disorder	20	13,824	9,982	
Adjusted diagnosis				
Dysthymia	7	12,300	8,200	
GAD	68	11,077	10,453	P = 0.03
Panic disorder	64	9,260	9,668	
Cothymia	71	15,135	22,524	

Reproduced from Knerer et al., (2005) with permission from John Wiley & Sons.

a recurrent disorder – were the three elements contributing most to costs at 12 years (Knerer et al., 2005). Similarly, patients with general neurotic syndrome were more likely to use specialist mental health services than patients without the syndrome.

6.3 Main Outcome Findings at 12 Years

At 12 years, an interim point in the follow-up study, we wished to examine the progress of each patient in the 10-year interval since their last face-to-face contact. As the primary outcome for this occasion, we chose the Neurotic Disorder Outcome Scale (NDOS) (Table 6.4), as this was deliberately created to cover all mental pathology over this time period.

The main results in Table 6.5 showed little difference in the demographic variables and treatment groups – but with higher scores (i.e., worse outcomes) for patients with cothymia (P = 0.011); for those who scored high on global psychopathology, anxiety, and depression scales at baseline; and in those with personality disturbance (P < 0.001) – with increasing NDOS scores with higher levels of severity (Figure 6.1).

Personality disorder contributed most to the final model of the outcome analysis created by Tony Johnson at the MRC Biostatistics Unit in Cambridge (Table 6.6). It was of interest that in this analysis the differences in scores on the observer-rated depression scale (MADRS) did not quite reach significance whereas the HADS-D was the strongest predictor.

Table 6.4 Neurotic Disorder Outcome Scale [NDOS]

1	More than one year with any of the following disorders: GAD, DYS, MDE, Ag, PAG, Ob, SOP
2	Developed alcohol dependence syndrome (DSM or ICD criteria)
3	Developed organic brain disorder (ICD F04-06) or DSM amnestic disorder (294) but excluding dementia
4	Follow-up SFQ score of 10 or greater
5	Subsequent disorder within the schizophrenia group (including delusional disorder) (F20-29-ICD-10 and 293, 295, 297, and 298 in DSM-IV)
6	More than 70% of follow-up with diagnosis equivalent to or more serious than original neurotic diagnosis (i.e., GAD, DYS, PAG, Ag, Ob, MDE, MEL, SOP)
7	Subsequent MDE or agoraphobia (any type) of more than two years' duration
8	More than four episodes of MDE (including MEL) during follow-up
9	Unnatural death (including accidental death, open verdict, and suicide)
10	Admitted to psychiatric hospital during follow-up
TOTAL	

Total score of 0–10 based on score of 1 for each of the 10 items
Key: GAD = generalised anxiety disorder, DYS = dysthymic disorder, MDE = major depressive episode, Ag = agoraphobia, PAG = agoraphobia with panic, Ob = obsessive-compulsive disorder, SOP = social phobia, MEL = melancholia

Table 6.5 Relationship between baseline characteristics and outcome as measured by the Neurotic Disorder Outcome Scale (NDOS) over 12 years in 193 patients

	Mean NDOS score (SD) with 95% CI for comparisons in brackets	F value	Significance (P)
Initial randomised treatment			
Drug therapy (n = 77)	1.3 (1.6)	0.2	0.62 (ns)
CBT (n = 77)	2.1 (1.7) (−0.62 to 0.37)	0.8	0.38 (ns)
Self-help (n = 39)	1.9 (1.9) (−0.88 to 0.33)		
Marital status			
Married/cohabiting n = 80	1.9 (1.7)	2.8	P = 0.095
Single n = 60	2.4 (1.9) (−0.07 to 0.97)		
Separated/divorced/widowed n = 53	2.2 (1.6) 0.02 (−0.53 to 0.56)		
Revised diagnosis			
Dysthymia n = 5	(1.9)	6.5	P = 0.011
GAD n = 64	1.8 (1.5)		
Panic disorder n = 57	1.8 (1.7)		
Mixed anxiety-depression (cothymia) n = 67	2.6 (1.8) 0.65 (0.15 to 1.16)		
Total psychopathology (CPRS)			
Score 0–16 n = 45	1.9 (1.8) 0.057 (0.028 to 0.086)	14.9	P<0.001
17–21 n = 54	1.5 (1.4)		
22–28 n = 49	2.5 (1.6)		
≥29 n = 45	2.7 (1.9)		
Observer-rated anxiety (BAS)			
Score 0–15 n = 48	1.9 (1.7) 0.045 (0.011 to 0.079)	6.8	P = 0.011
16–19 n = 50	1.5 (1.5)		
20–25 n = 51	2.5 (1.8)		
≥ 26+ n = 44	2.7 (1.8)		

Table 6.5 (cont.)

Observer-rated depression (MADRS)		
Score 0–15 n = 55	1.8 (1.7) 0.028 (0.002 to 0.058)	3.4	P = 0.07
16–19 n = 43	2.1 (1.8)		
20–25 n = 47	2.3 (1.6)		
≥ 26 n = 48	2.4 (1.8)		
Self-rated anxiety (HADS-A)			
Score 0–8 n = 21	1.8 (1.8) 0.069 (0.001 to 0.14) 1.8 (1.7)	4.0	P = 0.049
9–12 n = 36	2.2 (1.7)		
13–15 n = 61	2.4 (1.8)		
16–22 n = 75			
Self-rated depression (HADS-D)			
Score 0–8 n = 68	1.5 (1.4) 0.13 (0.07–0.18)	23.1	P < 0.001
9–12 n = 57	2.1 (1.7)		
13–15 n = 44	2.6 (1.8)		
16–22 n = 24	3.1 (1.8)		
Personality status			
No pers dys n = 84	1.7 (1.4) 0.50 (0.28 – 0.72)	19.8	P < 0.001
Pers diff n = 39	2.1 (2.0)		
Mild p dis n = 50	2.3 (1.7)		
Md/sev p dis n = 20	3.7 (1.4)		

Table 6.6 Final model showing the elements contributing most to clinical outcome at 12 years

Variable	Regression coefficient (95%CL)	Cumulative percentage of variation explained
Intercept	0.36 (−0.26, 0.97)	
HADS depression	0.11 (0.06, 0.17)	10.8
Personality status	0.42 (0.20, 0.63)	16.9
Single marital status	0.52 (0.05, 1.00)	18.9

This table shows the final model including the three baseline variables; excluding single marital status, which produces only minor changes in the other two regression coefficients (and their 95% confidence limits). The model suggests that, on average, a change of one category in NDOS score results from a change of 9 units on the HADS depression score, and a change of 2.5 'units' in personality status.

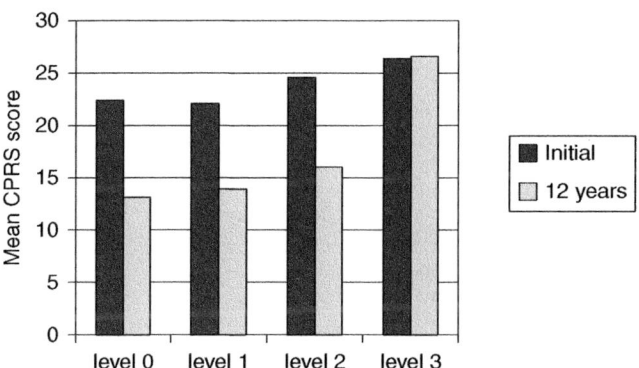

Figure 6.1 Effect of personality status on global symptomatology (measured by the Comprehensive Psychopathological Rating Scale (CPRS) at baseline and 12 years)
Personality severity code: level 0 = no personality disorder; level 1 = personality difficulty; level 2 = simple personality disorder; level 3 = diffuse or complex personality disorder

6.4 Social Function

6.4.1 Analysis of Data

There were two main aims in the analyses of social function. The first was to examine if there was any relationship between the initial personality ratings and social function at 12 years. The second was to determine the associations of the other 18 clinical and demographic variables with social function.

6.5 Findings – First Aim

Of the total number of patients, 187 (84 per cent) completed the Social Functioning Questionnaire (SFQ) at 12 years. The mean SFQ score in those seen was 8.0, with significantly lower mean scores for those with no personality disorder at baseline using both the original categorical model (no personality disorder (n = 113) (mean SFQ 6.8, SD 4.9), compared with those with cluster A (n = 11) (mean SFQ 11.6, SD 4.0), cluster B (n = 29)(mean SFQ 9.0, SD 5.8), and cluster C (n = 24) personality disorders (mean SFQ 10.4, SD 6.1, (F = 5.9, df 3,173; P < 0.001).

6.6 Findings – Second Aim

At 12 years, the most common ICD-10 personality disorders were avoidant (n = 24), paranoid (n = 17), dependent (n = 9), and antisocial (n = 8). The results of the first stage of the univariate regression analysis are shown in Table 6.7. Those with little or no personality disturbance, of higher social class, those with single diagnoses rather than cothymia, those ever married, and those with lower levels of anxiety and depression at baseline, all had better social function at 12 years than others. The 18 variables (Table 6.7) were then included in a multiple linear regression analysis predicting SFQ scores at 12 years.

The results at 12 years (Table 6.8) generally support the hypothesis that personality disorder and the general neurotic syndrome are associated with long-term social dysfunction. This is not a trivial finding. Some look on diagnosis, particularly of

Table 6.7 Relationship between other baseline variables and outcome in terms of social function (SFQ) at 12 years

Baseline variable	N	SF score [mean (SD)]	Regression coefficient (95% CL)	F (P)	%
Gender					
Male	56	8.8 (4.6)			
Female	121	7.6 (5.7)	−1.27 (−2.96, 0.43)	2.1 (0.14)	1.2
Age group (years)					
<30	59	8.9 (6.0)	−0.53 (−1.21, 0.16)	2.3 (0.13)	1.3
30–44	81	7.7 (5.1)			
45+	37	7.1 (4.9)			
Social class					
1, 2	24	6.3 (4.5)	1.18 (0.39, 1.96)	8.7 (0.007)	4.7
3	38	6.6 (4.5)			
4	67	8.2 (5.6)			
5	48	9.5 (5.7)			

Table 6.7 (cont.)

Baseline variable	N	SF score [mean (SD)]	Regression coefficient (95% CL)	F (P)	%
Marital status					
Single	56	9.9 (5.5)			
Married/cohabiting	73	6.8 (5.2)	2.91 (1.26, 4.57)	11.9 (<0.001)	6.4
Separated/divorced/widowed	48	7.4 (4.9)	−0.80 (−2.58, 0.99)	0.8 (0.38)	0.4
Initial randomised treatment					
Drug therapy	71	8.0 (5.2)			
CBT	71	8.0 (5.5)	0.15 (−1.47, 1.77)	0.0 (0.90)	<0.1
Self-help	35	7.7 (5.8)	−0.37 (−2.37, 1.62)	0.1 (0.72)	<0.1
Initial diagnosis					
GAD	60	7.5 (5.1)	−0.74 (−2.41, 0.94)		
Dysthymia	51	9.8 (5.0)		0.8 (0.39)	0.4
Panic disorder	66	7.0 (5.6)	−1.57 (−3.20, 0.06)	3.6 (0.058)	2.0
Original episode					
New	119	7.4 (5.4)	1.55 (−0.12, 3.23)	3.3 (0.069)	1.9
Recurrence	58	9.0 (5.2)			
Total psychopathology (CPRS)					
0–16	41	7.6 (5.8)	0.18 (0.08, 0.28)	13.1 (<0.001)	7.0
17–21	49	5.6 (4.4)			
22–28	45	8.3 (5.2)			
29+	42	10.6 (5.0)			
Observer rated depression (MADRS)					
0–15	50	6.8 (5.1)	0.15 (0.05, 0.25)	9.2 (0.002)	5.0
16–19	40	6.6 (5.3)			
20–25	43	8.4 (5.3)			
26+	44	10.0 (5.4)			
Observer rated anxiety (BAS)					
0–15	43	7.6 (5.2)	0.11 (0.0+, 0.22)	3.9 (0.049)	2.2
16–19	47	6.4 (4.7)			
20–25	46	8.6 (5.9)			
26+	41	9.3 (5.4)			

Table 6.7 (cont.)

Baseline variable	N	SF score [mean (SD)]	Regression coefficient (95% CL)	F (P)	%
Initial comorbidity					
Dysthymia	4	13.3 (2.9)	2.79 (1.16, 4.42)	11.3 (<0.001)	6.1
GAD	60	7.5 (5.1)			
Panic disorder	53	6.0 (4.7)			
Mixed (cothymia)	60	9.8 (5.6)			
General Neurotic Syndrome					
Absent	84	6.9 (5.2)			
Present	93	8.9 (5.4)	2.02 (0.45, 3.58)	6.4 (0.012)	3.5
Self-rated anxiety (HADS-A)					
0–8	18	7.7 (5.6)	0.23 (0.0+, 0.46)	4.0 (0.046)	2.2
9–12	33	6.4 (4.2)			
13–15	56	7.3 (4.9)			
16–22	70	9.3 (6.0)			
Self-rated depression (HADS-D)					
0–8	64	5.9 (4.5)	0.48 (0.30, 0.65)	28.7 (<0.001)	14.1
9–12	53	7.4 (5.1)			
13–15	39	10.0 (5.4)			
16–22	21	11.8 (5.3)			

From Seivewright, Tyrer & Johnson, 2004 (with kind permission of John Wiley & Sons).
The table shows the number of subjects in each category n; regression coefficient (95% confidence interval) from a simple (univariate) linear regression; the associated F-statistic on 1 and 175 df, and its P-value; and the percentage of variation (%) in Social Function scale score explained by the baseline covariate. The regression coefficient for age is *per decade*). Personality coding follows Tyrer and Johnson (1996) with 0 = no personality disorder, 1 = personality difficulty, 2 = simple personality disorder, 3 = diffuse (complex) personality disorder.

common mental disorders, as an unnecessary exercise as the essential point of presentation is to communicate distress. But if distress, as recorded in the form of social function, is higher in some populations than others then it is useful to diagnose these separately. The findings also show that although personality functioning may change, its baseline impact on long-term social function does not, and, together with the severity of self-rated depression and marital status, it was a key predictor of social function at 12 years.

Table 6.8 Final model of variables predicting social functioning score at 12 years in 177 patients

Variable	Regression coefficient (95% CI)	Cumulative percentage of variation explained
Intercept	0.83 (−1.09, 2.74)	
HADS depression	2.90 (1.44, 4.34)	14.1
Single marital status	0.81 (0.12, 1.49)	21.1
Personality status	1.24 (0.58, 1.91)	27.7
Social class	0.41 (0.25, 0.58)	29.9

From Seivewright et al., 2004 (with kind permission of John Wiley & Sons).

6.7 Interpretation of Results

Not all the results at 12 years are presented in this chapter and the concentration on social function and the NDOS scale has limitations, the main one being that it is not an established scale and therefore is not likely to be used by others. But it was ideal for examining the outcome of the general neurotic syndrome. The syndrome, if it develops further from its combined anxiety and depressive components, will extend into other (neurotic) diagnostic categories such as more severe depression, agoraphobia, social anxiety, and addictive disorders (see Chapter 1). There are even some who argue that the prolonged stress of such syndromes can lead to early dementia (evidence not strong so not cited here) and so organic states are also included in the scale.

The NDOS and economic evidence support the conclusions of the earlier results in the Nottingham Study and add some more layers to the argument that the general neurotic syndrome is an important condition. In summary, the 12-year findings show the GNS and its linked component of personality disorder are associated with:

(i)   higher service costs,

(ii) a worse outcome than other diagnoses, and

(iii) poorer social function than other conditions.

The data from the initial trial onwards all point towards the general neurotic syndrome having all the status of a good diagnosis.

The Last Phase

Chapter

7

The Last Phase
The General Neurotic Syndrome
after 30 Years

It is never too late to do a long-term follow-up study. Through long-term follow-up, a full knowledge of tardive dyskinesia, a condition once thought to be permanent, has illustrated that this is far from the case (e.g., Cavallaro et al., 1993). However, there is bound to be a loss of people to contact when you study follow-up at 30 years. The common word for this is attrition – 'the gradual reduction in the number of people who are involved in a study that is achieved by not replacing those who leave'. I have always found this word to be a somewhat euphemistic one; the usual cause of attrition is death. In the case of cancer studies, death (mortality) is the primary outcome in most cases. With the general neurotic syndrome, early death is clearly an important outcome, but mental health at follow-up is more so. Following the advice of Sir Richard Doll (see Chapter 3), we decided at this point to choose the dichotomous outcome of the absence or presence of one of the main DSM diagnoses. The very minor diagnoses such as simple phobia and adjustment disorders were not included here. This choice can always be criticised as it is seen to be made at a single point in time. But this is not exactly true. Most other diagnoses within the neurotic spectrum have a long duration; they may come and go but they do not disappear entirely. Our expectation was therefore that if there was no DSM diagnosis present at 30 years then the patient could be regarded as mentally well.

There were other problems to overcome at 30 years. The Data Protection Act has made it impossible to carry out studies in the NHS without approval from NHS Digital, the organisation that holds all the relevant data, but it will only release the data after you have overcome more hurdles than exist in the Grand National. This is not a complaint, but it does lead to a tremendous amount of delay. We also recognised that cold-calling would be essential at 30 years if patients do not respond to the initial letters sent to their putative addresses. Fortunately, with the assistance of colleagues at the Northampton Research Ethics Committee, we were able to have cold calling approved using the same approach as we did at 12 years.

7.1 Procedure Used in 30-Year Follow-Up

Exactly the same procedure was used at 30 years as at 12 years, but with an additional measure of personality, that of personality strengths (rarely recorded in personality disorder research). The measure was a new one that examined each of the 24 variables in the Personality Assessment Schedule from a different angle.

So, for example, the opposite of worthlessness in the Personality Assessment Schedule-Strengths Version (PAS-SV) is self-confidence. Here are two questions from the schedule:

Sometimes belief in your own worth can be of help in overcoming problems in life. Do you have this belief in your worth?
Some people have such self-confidence that they achieve success in life. Has self-confidence helped you in any way?

There are several limitations to the PAS-SV. It was created in 1983 at the time of the start of the Nottingham Study but was never properly tested. It includes several words that do not yet exist – 'placatorianess' is the ability to be placatory but there is

Table 7.1 The 24 components of the Personality Assessment Schedule (PAS) and the Personality Assessment Schedule-Strengths Version (PAS-SV)

PAS	PAS-SV
Pessimism	Prudence
Worthlessness	Self-confidence
Optimism	Certainty
Lability	Stability
Anxiousness	Stress steadiness
Suspiciousness	Openness
Introspection	Decisiveness
Shyness	Social competence
Aloofness	Gregariousness
Sensitivity	Ruthlessness
Vulnerability	Toughness
Irritability	Equanimity
Impulsivity	Carefulness
Aggression	Placatorianess
Callousness	Empathicness
Irresponsibility	High responsibility
Childishness	Maturity
Resourcelessness	Positive drive (resourcefulness)
Dependence	Independence
Submissiveness	Dominance
Conscientiousness	Opportunism
Rigidity	Adaptability
Eccentricity	Conformity
Hypochondriasis	Positive healthiness

no equivalent in the English language. The PAS-SV had still not been tested by the time of follow-up but my wife, Helen, felt it must be included at the 30-year point as it was a relevant measure – she was right. The PAS-SV also includes one of the important components of the so-called Big Five, the key five traits underlying personality (Costa and McCrae, 1992). 'Openness to experience' is one of the Big Five but does not appear in any grouping of personality disorder traits. Why not? Because it is a personality strength, not a handicap.

It is also quite possible for the same individual to score high on both the PAS and the PAS-SV, usually at different times, even though they appear to be contradictory. One of the early patients in the Nottingham Study had a very poor relationship with her husband and found him 'utterly boring'. She told me she had tried to kill him by putting rat poison in his evening meal but he recognised the taste was odd and refused to eat it. She was annoyed by her failure here and in her discussion with me she justified her actions along the lines of 'his life was pretty useless and there was not much point in him staying alive'. Later on in the study he became ill (for reasons quite unconnected with his wife's behaviour) and eventually died. During the time of his last illness, she was very assiduous in looking after him, being aware of and responding to all his needs, and seemed to have forgotten entirely about the rat poison episode. So she could score highly on being both callous and empathic.

The PAS-SV was administered to all the patients seen at 30 years. The results were subjected to factor analysis, the standard method of determining how these 24 variables group together. Five clear factors emerged (Table 7.2)(Yang, Tyrer, and Tyrer, 2022). The impact of the PAS-SV ratings is discussed in Section 7.7; it needs more context.

Table 7.2 Factor analysis of the Personality Assessment Schedule-Strengths Version (PAS-SV)

Factor	Variance explained %	Key items	PAS-SV traits	Collective name
1	17.0	12, 14, 15, 16, 17	equanimity, placatorianess, empathicness, high positive responsibility, maturity	Forceful/ reliable
2	31.5	1, 2, 3, 4, 5, 18, 19	prudence, self-confidence, certainty, stability, stress steadiness, positive drive, independence	Tough mindedness
3	44.5	6, 8, 9, 21, 22	openness, social competence, gregariousness, opportunism, adaptability	Sociability and personal independence
4	56.7	7, 11, 13, 23, 24	decisiveness, toughness, carefulness, conformity, positive healthiness	Cautiousness
5	65.9	10, 20	ruthlessness, dominance	Focused discernment

7.2 Results of 30-Year Assessments

Fewer patients were assessed at 30 years. The complete data from baseline onwards are shown in Figure 7.1.

7.3 Deaths

There were 71 deaths recorded during the 30 years; 36 (34.3% of those with the general neurotic syndrome) and 35 (34.0% of those without the syndrome). This was a negligible difference ($\chi^2 = 0.009$; df 1, P = 0.92). So, despite all the accumulating negative data from other parts of the study, there was no evidence of earlier mortality in this condition.

Personality status showed a trend in favour of earlier death in more severely personality disordered patients when these were studied by severity status alone, but those with no personality dysfunction at baseline died earlier (Table 7.3). Analysis of cause of death showed no particular associations; and when a multivariate linear regression model was used to estimate effects of the severity of personality disorder on the lifespan of patients with adjustment for clinical diagnosis at baseline, gender, and age of patients at the point of randomisation to the study, the findings showed that earlier death was more associated with initial clinical diagnosis than personality (Table 7.3) (Tyrer, Tyrer, and Yang, 2021).

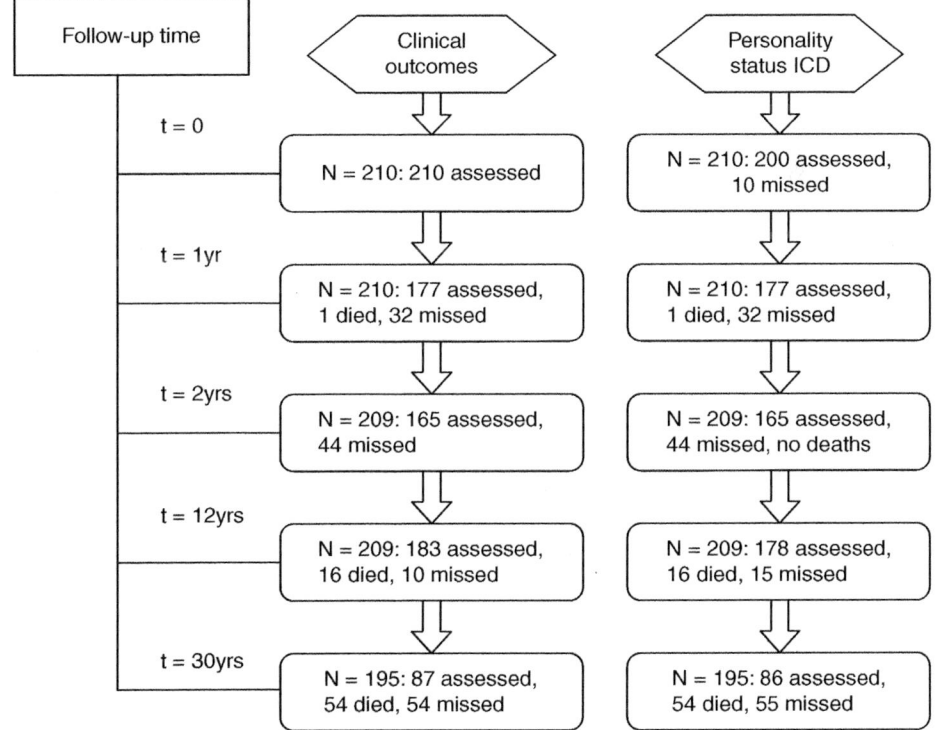

Figure 7.1 Flow chart of missing individuals for outcome assessments by follow-up time point

Table 7.3 Distribution of deaths in the Nottingham Study by personality status

PD diagnosis	Patients at baseline	Death 30 years later (%)
No personality dysfunction (level 0)	87	38 (43.7)
Personality difficulty (level 1)	40	11 (27.5)
Mild personality disorder (level 2)	50	14 (28.0)
Moderate (level 3) & severe personality disorder (level 4)	23	8 (34.8)
Missing data at baseline	10	
All	210	71 (35.5)

$\chi^2 = 4.853$, df = 3, P = 0.18

7.4 Clinical Outcomes

7.4.1 DSM Status at 30 Years

The results of the primary outcome (DSM status) are shown in Table 7.4. These are important in the context of the general neurotic syndrome as they help to refine my original hypothesis in Chapter 1: 'If a person has both anxiety and depressive symptoms and some personality disturbance the diagnosis of the general neurotic syndrome is the best way of defining the problem.' The change is a small one but excludes panic from the diagnostic framework of the syndrome, provided it is not associated with depressive symptoms. The data in the original trial suggested panic was just a more severe form of generalised anxiety (see Figure 4.1) but the data from 12 years onwards show differences that are far from trivial and suggest that panic disorder has the best outcome of the anxious depressive group of disorders (provided it is not combined with depressive symptoms).

7.5 Psychopathology and Influence of the General Neurotic Syndrome over 12 and 30 Years

The results by diagnosis were consistent with previous findings. Patients with panic had total psychopathology scores 30% lower than those with cothymia, and those with moderate/severe personality disorder had scores nearly twice as high as those with no personality disorder (Table 7.5).

The outcome by GNS status is shown in Tables 7.6 and 7.7, and here it is useful to show the data at both 12 and 30 years. The findings show little change over the 18-year period between assessments, with only the HADS-D depression self-rating deviating from its mean ratings at 12 years to show some improvement by 30 years, but the overall differences over both time periods showed increasing pathology for all measures.

Social function in patients with baseline positive GNS findings was more than 50% worse than in those without the syndrome (Table 7.7). The NDOS ratings were very similar.

Table 7.4 Formal psychiatric diagnosis (DSM) at long-term follow-up points

Condition at baseline	12th year			30th year			Joint and adjusted estimate[b]	
	N	DSM+, %	P[a]	N	DSM+, %	P[a]	AOR (95% CI)	P
GNS status			0.024			0.170		0.0074
GNS < 6	121	55.4		60	45.0		(Ref)	
GNS ≥ 6	65	72.3		28	60.7		2.25 (1.24–4.08)	
DSM-III			0.609			0.027		
GAD	63	57.1		26	57.7		(Ref)	
Panic	55	60.0		32	31.3		0.76 (0.40–1.47)	0.422
Cothymia	64	65.6		30	63.3		1.41 (0.74–2.72)	0.299
ICD-11 status			0.027			0.061		
No PD	76	56.6		34	34.3		(Ref)	
PD difficulty	39	48.7		16	56.3		0.90 (0.45–1.84)	0.784
Mild PD	45	75.6		24	58.3		2.22 (1.10–4.47)	0.026
Moderate & severe PD	21	76.2		12	75.0		2.88 (1.10–7.56)	0.031

[a] Based on Chi-square test.
AOR = Odds ratio of joint outcome for both 12 and 30 years adjusted for age and sex.

Table 7.5 Total psychopathology scores (CPRS) at long-term follow-up points

Condition at baseline		12th year		30th year	Joint and adjusted estimate[b]
	N	Adjusted[a] Mean (95% CI)	N	Adjusted[a] Mean (95% CI)	Mean difference (SE): P
Diagnoses					
GAD	62	14.63 (11.48–17.78)	26	16.41 (11.49–21.34)	(Ref)
Panic	54	13.49 (10.28–16.70)	32	15.48 (10.89–20.07)	−1.04 (1.88): 0.578
Cothymia	62	18.77 (15.46–22.08)	29	20.81 (15.97–25.65)	4.20 (1.81): 0.021
Overall P		0.016		0.199	0.011
ICD-11 status					
No PD	75	12.40 (9.41–15.39)	35	13.37 (9.02–17.72)	(Ref)
PD difficulty	39	13.22 (9.54–16.90)	16	19.31 (13.16–25.46)	1.09 (1.98): 0.571
Mild PD	43	19.23 (15.80–22.66)	24	18.19 (13.14–23.24)	6.59 (1.89): 0.00048
Moderate & severe PD	21	17.48 (12.79–22.17)	12	23.55 (16.55–30.55)	5.60 (2.45): 0.022
Overall P		0.0024		0.054	0.0018

[a] Adjusted for age and sex, and conditional on measures of other time points. [b] Joint outcome of 12 and 30 years, adjusted for age and sex and conditional on measures of other time points. Note differences at 30 years need to be greater than at 12 years to achieve significance.

Table 7.6 Clinical outcome by GNS status at long-term follow-up points and mean CPRS scores

Outcome		12th year		30th	Joint and adjusted estimate[b]
CPRS	N	Adjusted[a] Mean (95% CI)	N	Adjusted[a] Mean (95% CI)	Mean difference (SE): P
GNS < 6	119	13.35 (10.96–15.74)	59	14.65 (11.23–18.05)	(Ref)
GNS ≥ 6	64	19.56 (16.44–22.68)	28	23.14 (18.40–27.88)	6.44 (1.52): 0.000022
P		0.00010		0.0019	
HADS-A					
GNS < 6	119	7.89 (6.73–9.05)	59	8.11 (6.53–9.69)	(Ref)
GNS ≥ 6	63	11.49 (9.97–13.01)	28	10.37 (8.19–12.55)	3.37 (0.70): 0.0000
P		0.0000		0.071	
HADS-D					
GNS < 6	119	6.27 (5.03–7.51)	59	6.46 (4.91–8.01)	(Ref)
GNS ≥ 6	63	8.53 (6.92–10.14)	28	7.83 (5.71–9.95)	2.11 (0.73): 0.0039
P		0.0060		0.249	
BAS					
GNS < 6	119	9.59 (7.70–11.48)	59	10.13 (7.56–12.70)	(Ref)
GNS ≥ 6	64	14.55 (12.09–17.01)	28	14.98 (11.43–18.53)	5.00 (1.15): 0.000014
P		0.000058		0.017	

Table 7.6 (cont.)

Outcome					Joint and adjusted estimate[b]
		12th year		**30th**	
CPRS	**N**	**Adjusted[a] Mean (95% CI)**	**N**	**Adjusted[a] Mean (95% CI)**	**Mean difference (SE): P**
MADRS					
GNS < 6	**119**	11.24 (8.85–13.63)	**59**	10.72 (7.43–14.01)	(Ref)
GNS ≥ 6	**64**	16.34 (13.21–19.47)	**28**	16.70 (12.11–21.29)	5.27 (1.42): 0.00020
P		0.0024		0.025	

[a] Adjusted for age and sex, and conditional on measures of other time points. [b] Joint outcome of 12 and 30 years, adjusted for age and sex, and conditional on measures of other time points.

Table 7.7 Social function – measured by the Social Functioning Questionnaire (SFQ) and the Neurotic Disorder Outcome Scale (NDOS) at long-term follow-up points

Outcome variable	**12th year unadjusted**		**30th year unadjusted**		**Joint and adjusted estimate[a]**	
	N: Mean (SD)	**P**	**N: Mean (SD)**	**P**	**Mean difference (95% CI)**	**P**
SFQ		0.006		0.005		
GNS < 6	119: 7.01 (5.23)		59: 6.80 (5.31)		(Ref)	
GNS≥ 6	64: 9.27 (5.38)		28: 10.32 (5.49)		3.04 (1.56–4.52)	0.000
NDOS		0.075		0.045		
GNS < 6	119: 1.97 (1.78)		60: 1.42 (2.09)		(Ref)	
GNS ≥ 6	65: 2.45 (1.71)		28: 2.50 (2.40)		0.64 (0.12–1.16)	0.016
SFQ		0.077		0.033		
GAD	63: 7.49 (5.09)		26: 8.15 (6.18)		(Ref)	
Panic	54: 5.91 (4.70)		32: 5.88 (5.76)		−1.84 (−3.55−−0.13)	0.034
Cothymia	62: 9.53 (5.72)		29: 9.93 (5.26)		2.11 (0.44–3.78)	0.014
NDOS		0.056		0.145		
GAD	63: 1.89 (1.55)		26: 1.58 (2.14)		(Ref)	
Panic	54: 1.87 (1.72)		32: 1.22 (2.18)		−0.64 (−0.66−0.53)	0.824
Cothymia	63: 2.52 (1.83)		30: 2.30 (2.18)		0.71 (0.13–1.29)	0.016
SFQ		0.000		0.028		
No PD	75: 6.27 (4.42)		35: 6.29 (4.59)		(Ref)	
PD difficulty	39: 7.82 (5.58)		15: 8.87 (6.28)		1.54 (−0.30–3.38)	0.102
Mild PD	43: 9.56 (5.70)		24: 8.17 (5.78)		2.66 (0.90–4.42)	0.031
Moderate & severe PD	21: 10.86 (5.51)		12: 11.67 (5.40)		4.51 (2.26–6.75)	0.000
NDOS		0.006		0.079		
No PD	75: 1.75 (1.46)		35: 1.31 (2.04)		(Ref)	
PD difficulty	39: 2.03 (2.01)		16: 1.69 (2.27)		0.24 (−0.41–0.88)	0.476
Mild PD	44: 2.61 (1.79)		24: 1.79 (2.19)		0.76 (0.14–1.37)	0.016
Moderate & severe PD	21: 3.00 (1.82)		12: 3.25 (2.49)		1.25 (0.45–2.05)	0.0065

[a] Estimation by bivariate linear models and adjusted for age and sex.

7.6 Treatments Received by GNS Status

In Table 7.8 the main treatments received by the patients separated by their GNS status are summarised over the follow-up periods at 12 and 30 years. The most striking findings are that in those who were GNS positive at baseline; there were (1) a greater number of GP contacts, (2) longer duration of day care, and (3) greater psychotropic drug consumption.

7.7 Influence of Personality Strengths

The results of the personality strengths analysis are of great interest but because they constitute a new type of assessment there are no data by which they can be compared. Female patients had somewhat greater strength scores than males, especially on cautiousness; cothymic patients had lower scores on all measures (P = 0.02), but, interestingly, GNS positive patients only had significantly lower scores on emotional toughness. Personality disorder, not unexpectedly, was associated with lower strength scores in an incremental association with severity. The CPRS scores at baseline showed indications

Table 7.8 Differences in treatment and service contacts between patients with or without the general neurotic syndrome

0–12 years	GNS (0–4) N: Mean ± SD	GNS (5–6) N: Mean ± SD	GNS (≥6) N: Mean ± SD	Sig level	Linear trend
No. of GP/OP appts for psych illness	89: 27.9 ± 26.0	29: 26.8 ± 26.3	61: 38.3 ± 32.3	**0.050**	**0.024**
No. of GP/OP appts for non-psych illness	90: 60.6 ± 42.9	29: 58.6 ± 38.3	61: 68.8 ± 42.5	0.392	0.211
Length of day care (weeks)	90: 2.00 ± 6.6	29: 4.28 ± 14.7	61: 8.13 ± 15.0	**0.004**	**0.002**
Weeks of non-psych hospitalisation	90: 1.29 ± 2.1	29: 1.41 ± 1.9	61: 1.41 ± 2.0	0.608	0.385
Weeks of psych hospitalisation	90: 0.67 ± 2.1	29: 0.17 ± 0.9	61: 1.36 ± 5.4	0.359	0.729
No. of admission	90: 1.83 ± 2.8	29: 1.55 ± 2.4	61: 2.08 ± 2.7	0.638	0.405
Months with no psychotropic medication	96: 113.4 ± 39.7	31: 112.6 ± 42.6	66: 91.7 ± 50.9	**0.012**	**0.004**
0–30 years					
Months with no psychotropic medication	41: 293.1 ± 109.1	18: 265.4 ± 104.8	27:209.5 ± 141.2	**0.008**	**0.004**

AOR = adjusted odds ratio.
For scale measures, ANOVA was performed based on logarithm transformed scale and so was the linearity test.
For the categorical measures, Fisher's exact test was used to provide the p-values for both difference and linearity.

Table 7.3 Personality strengths by baseline characteristics of patients

Characteristics	PASP traits					
	Forcefulness	Emotional toughness	Cautiousness	Independence	Discernment	Total
Sex: N						
Female: 63	17.8 ± 7.2	19.6 ± 9.5	14.8 ± 7.2	13.3 ± 6.8	4.5 ± 3.1	70.0 ± 29.5
Male: 26	15.2 ± 6.8	17.7 ± 8.8	11.7 ± 6.5	13.0 ± 6.5	3.8 ± 3.1	61.4 ± 26.9
P-value	0.121	0.386	0.061	0.851	0.321	0.202
DSM Diag.						
Dys: 1	8 ± n/a	11.0 ± n/a	7.0 ± n/a	12.0 ± n/a	2.0 ± n/a	40.0 ± n/a
GAD: 26	18.1 ± 7.5	20.6 ± 9.1	13.7 ± 8.3	14.5 ± 7.2	3.8 ± 3.3	70.7 ± 31.6
Panic: 32	19.6 ± 5.7	20.8 ± 10.1	16.8 ± 6.5	14.6 ± 6.5	5.1 ± 3.1	76.9 ± 26.9
Cothymia: 30	13.8 ± 7.1	16.0 ± 8.1	11.3 ± 5.7	10.7 ± 5.9	3.9 ± 2.9	55.7 ± 24.8
P-value	**0.004**	0.121	**0.016**	0.086	0.289	**0.020**
GNS score						
< 4: 42	17.4 ± 7.3	20.9 ± 9.1	14.1 ± 7.2	14.1 ± 6.7	4.0 ± 3.2	71.0 ± 28.8
4–5: 18	19.3 ± 7.1	20.6 ± 10.0	14.6 ± 7.3	13.6 ± 7.5	5.3 ± 2.9	73.5 ± 29.8
≥ 6: 28	15.1 ± 7.0	15.4 ± 8.5	12.1 ± 6.8	11.7 ± 6.2	4.0 ± 3.1	58.4 ± 27.8
P-value	0.147	**0.039**	0.330	0.323	0.296	0.127
PD status						
None: 35	20.2 ± 6.2	21.4 ± 8.6	16.2 ± 6.9	15.3 ± 6.2	4.9 ± 3.0	80.0 ± 26.5
Difficulty: 16	16.8 ± 7.6	16.6 ± 10.2	11.2 ± 8.2	11.2 ± 7.1	4.1 ± 2.5	59.9 ± 32.3
Simple: 24	15.4 ± 6.9	19.4 ± 8.6	14.5 ± 6.1	13.4 ± 6.4	4.0 ± 3.3	66.8 ± 25.7
Moderate/severe: 12	11.5 ± 6.6	14.6 ± 10.4	8.6 ± 5.1	9.1 ± 6.4	3.0 ± 3.8	46.8 ± 27.3
P-value	**0.001**	0.109	**0.004**	**0.022**	0.282	**0.007**
CPRS score						
< 15: 15	17.4 ± 6.8	20.5 ± 8.9	14.2 ± 7.1	14.2 ± 6.2	2.8 ± 2.7	69.0 ± 26.7
15–25: 45	17.8 ± 7.4	20.5 ± 9.6	15.2 ± 7.8	13.8 ± 7.0	5.1 ± 3.0	72.4 ± 30.9
≥ 26: 27	15.6 ± 7.3	15.8 ± 8.6	11.1 ± 5.4	11.4 ± 6.5	3.7 ± 3.1	57.6 ± 25.6
P-value	0.460	0.093	0.060	0.278	**0.023**	0.109

PASP = positive personality traits from the Comprehensive Personality Assessment Scale (CPAS)

of lower strength scores with higher baseline pathology but the association was not strong.

Comparison of the data at 30 years showed very important differences. Suicide attempts were associated with few personality strengths, both for total scores and for each of the five main traits (Table 7.10). Those attending day centres also had low scores (but the numbers were small), and both social dysfunction (SFQ) and total psychopathology (CPRS) were much more marked in those with fewer personality strengths. Those with strong elements of forcefulness were more likely to be arrested and to be in custody (Table 7.10).

7.8 Synthesis of Findings

The study of a single syndrome, though unusual, over 30 years might be expected to yield a set of complex results and difficulties in interpretation. This may well be true at some levels, but at the level for justification of the general neurotic syndrome it is much easier. It is possible to state with some confidence that the syndrome is clinically useful and, dare I say it, valid, in the sense that it deserves to be studied further, rather than valid in the absolute sense.

The evidence from the 30 years of the Nottingham Study suggests the general neurotic syndrome differs from single depressive, anxious, and panic disorders in important (or at least non-trivial) ways:

(1) It is associated with greater symptomatology.
(2) It responds to treatment less well.
(3) It is associated with greater social dysfunction.
(4) It is associated with persistently worse clinical outcomes.
(5) It leads to greater service costs.
(6) It is associated with fewer personality strengths.

I will now examine each of these from the standpoint of a sceptical critic (as much as I am able to dissociate in that direction).

1   Greater Symptomatology

This is an easy win for the sceptic. The general neurotic syndrome comprises symptoms of both anxiety and depression and so is bound to have greater symptomatology than single symptom disorders. I will allow the sceptic to win this one.

2   Poor Response to Treatment

The general neurotic syndrome does not respond to conventional psychiatric treatment. This applies at every time point from 10 weeks onwards: the patients with the general neurotic syndrome fared less well than other patients. The late James Birley, another former president of the Royal College of Psychiatrists, used to quote among the many human rights that 'everyone should have the right to take part in a well-controlled randomised controlled trial'. Not only was he right but there is much good evidence that taking part in a good randomised trial in psychiatry is very good for your health, no matter what treatment you receive. This is even true when the treatments tested are no better than a placebo (Sanatinia et al., 2019). But even in the 10 weeks of the randomised trial, those with the general neurotic syndrome had worse outcomes than other groups, and these poorer outcomes were maintained over the whole 30-year period.

Table 7.10 Personality strength by characteristics of patients at 30-year follow-up

Characteristics	Forcefulness	Emotional toughness	Cautiousness	Independence	Discernment	Total
Suicide attempts: N						
None: 63	18.3 ± 6.8	20.9 ± 9.1	15.1 ± 7.1	14.7 ± 6.4	4.8 ± 3.2	73.8 ± 27.8
1–2 times: 12	13.9 ± 7.4	12.3 ± 5.3	11.1 ± 5.0	8.5 ± 5.1	3.0 ± 2.1	48.8 ± 19.1
3 times and more: 6	8.7 ± 3.8	10.3 ± 7.2	5.2 ± 3.4	5.8 ± 3.5	1.2 ± 1.5	31.2 ± 11.6
P-value	**0.001**	**0.000**	**0.001**	**0.000**	**0.006**	**0.000**
Social work contacts: N						
None: 79	17.7 ± 7.0	19.6 ± 9.3	14.3 ± 7.3	13.7 ± 6.6	4.3 ± 3.2	69.7 ± 28.7
1–5 times: 3	11.0 ± 3.5	11.3 ± 7.6	8.7 ± 5.9	8.0 ± 5.0	3.3 ± 1.5	42.3 ± 12.7
6 times and more: 7	12.9 ± 8.6	15.4 ± 8.9	11.7 ± 5.6	10.0 ± 7.3	3.6 ± 3.0	53.6 ± 28.9
P-value	0.076	0.180	0.289	0.141	0.701	0.112
Day centre care: N						
None: 85	17.5 ± 7.0	19.5 ± 9.2	14.2 ± 7.1	13.7 ± 6.4	4.4 ± 3.1	69.4 ± 28.2
Yes: 4	7.3 ± 3.5	10.0 ± 6.1	7.0 ± 3.7	2.8 ± 1.7	1.5 ± 1.7	28.5 ± 6.8
P-value	**0.004**	**0.046**	**0.047**	**0.001**	0.067	**0.005**
Arrested: N						
None: 80	17.6 ± 7.2	19.4 ± 9.5	14.3 ± 7.1	13.7 ± 6.7	4.5 ± 3.1	69.4 ± 29.1
Yes: 9	12.3 ± 5.0	16.1 ± 7.2	10.0 ± 6.3	9.7 ± 5.9	2.7 ± 2.3	50.8 ± 21.3
P-value	**0.036**	0.323	0.084	0.090	0.101	0.066
In custody: N						
None: 84	17.5 ± 7.1	19.5 ± 9.3	14.3 ± 7.2	13.5 ± 6.7	4.4 ± 3.1	69.2 ± 28.8
Yes: 5	10.0 ± 3.9	11.8 ± 6.2	7.4 ± 1.8	8.8 ± 4.0	2.0 ± 1.9	40.0 ± 10.1
P-value	**0.022**	0.074	**0.035**	0.127	0.091	**0.027**

Table 7.10 (cont.)

Characteristics	Forcefulness	Emotional toughness	Cautiousness	Independence	Discernment	Total
SFQ score: N						
< 4: 33	21.8 ± 5.7	25.8 ± 8.4	19.0 ± 5.8	18.2 ± 5.4	5.4 ± 3.3	90.2 ± 23.4
5–14: 42	15.2 ± 6.5	16.4 ± 6.8	11.8 ± 6.2	11.2 ± 5.5	4.0 ± 2.7	58.7 ± 22.2
≥ 15: 13	11.7 ± 5.8	11.2 ± 7.8	8.3 ± 5.4	7.8 ± 5.5	2.5 ± 2.8	41.5 ± 21.2
P-value	**0.000**	**0.000**	**0.000**	**0.000**	**0.012**	**0.000**
CPRS score						
< 15: 43	20.5 ± 6.7	25.0 ± 7.7	17.9 ± 5.7	17.3 ± 5.7	5.5 ± 3.1	86.2 ± 23.4
15–25: 21	15.5 ± 5.8	15.8 ± 7.0	11.7 ± 6.5	11.3 ± 5.1	3.0 ± 2.6	57.4 ± 22.0
≥ 26: 24	12.6 ± 6.0	11.6 ± 6.5	9.0 ± 6.2	7.9 ± 4.9	3.3 ± 2.7	44.4 ± 20.2
P-value	**0.000**	**0.000**	**0.000**	**0.000**	**0.001**	**0.000**

But the patients with the general neurotic syndrome were not neglected by services. They received more GP and outpatient contacts and more day care than other patients, and also many more psychotropic drugs (Table 7.8) (Tyrer et al., 2022). These treatments included more than 20 different psychotropic drugs, intensive psychological treatments ranging from analytical therapy, transactional analysis, cognitive behaviour therapy, and couple and group therapy (but none of the newer treatments for personality disorder), as well as more admissions to hospital. So they consulted more often, received more treatments, had more specialised secondary care, but apparently did not benefit. But the message is not all gloom. The conclusion should be 'a poor response to standard evidence-based treatments', but elsewhere there is a more positive message.

3   **Associated with Greater Social Dysfunction (see Table 7.7)**

4   **Associated with Persistently Worse Clinical Outcomes (see Table 7.6)**

5   **Leads to Greater Service Costs (see Table 6.3)**

6   **Associated with Fewer Personality Strengths (see Table 7.9)**

Chapter 8

Is the Notion of the General Neurotic Syndrome Useful?

In this last chapter, I want to write about the clinical implications of the general neurotic syndrome as a central part of neurosis. Clearly, I am biased, but I will try to give opposite arguments a fair airing too.

My starting point is a sentence from the ace nosologist, Bob Kendell; 'All our diagnostic terms are simply concepts, and the only fundamental question we can ask about them is whether they are useful concepts, and useful to whom?' (Kendell, 1991). This is the best riposte to those who decry the notion of diagnosis altogether. What it comes down to is utility. If the general neurotic syndrome is just a pimple on the side of common mental disorder that has no value except as an esoteric talking point, it is useless. I suggest a debate with six questions.

8.1 Does the General Neurotic Syndrome Add to the Understanding of Common Mental Illness?

To those who regard diagnosis in psychiatry as a pointless self-serving example of medical dominance, the notion of the general neurotic syndrome will just lead to eye-rolling and shaking of heads. I can see the sharing of annoyance on social media – yet another example of medical expansionism; creating a label in order to mask distress and normal human emotion.

A more common view in more informed circles is that the general neurotic syndrome, like almost all diagnoses in psychiatry, is just at the extreme end of the spectrum of common mental disorder and does not need separate demarcation. This comes back to the notion of usefulness. If the decisions made about the management of the general neurotic syndrome do not apply to other common mental disorders, then the diagnosis might be regarded as useful. The reasons why I think it is useful are expressed more fully here, and it also needs to be pointed out that the syndrome is not at an extreme of the spectrum of neurosis; it covers quite a large proportion.

It could also be said that comorbidity is all that is necessary to explain the syndrome. The reason why I think this is a mistake is that the term 'comorbidity', when properly used, describes the simultaneous presence of two separate disorders in the same person (Feinstein, 1970). The combination of anxiety, depression, and personality disturbance is not comorbidity; it is best expressed as consanguinity, manifestations of the same condition (Tyrer, 1996). But because personality is usually ignored in making the diagnosis, the general neurotic syndrome comes under the grouping described in Chapter 2, the Galenic syndromes, those conditions in which personality and clinical symptoms and behaviour are so closely intertwined that they have to be considered together. Now that the second axis of classification has been abandoned in the DSM classification, there has to be greater acknowledgement of the importance of personality in the description of these disorders.

My view here is not an isolated one. If we want to have a better understanding of mood and anxiety disorders, we have to take account of personality. This is particularly obvious when looking at the long-term outcomes of disorders. In Quinton et al.'s analysis of the 20-year follow-up of psychiatric disorder there was a strong plea for the recognition of personality as a key element of prediction: 'the results provide strong evidence for the value of a categorical diagnosis of personality disorder based on pervasive abnormalities in social functioning, and for a broad vision of such disorders into 'dramatic' and 'dependent/avoidant' types. Personality disorder proved to be a particularly strong predictor of the recurrence of depression' (Quinton et al., 1995, p. 321).

Michael Berk and an influential group of Australian and New Zealand colleagues have become very frustrated with the neglect of personality.

> We further argue for the benefit of adopting or incorporating a formulation-based approach that incorporates personality style and/or disorder. The use of personality and developmentally informed clinical formulations adds qualitative depth to clinical understanding. This is normative in some countries and settings, but not internationally. A formulation that includes personality would facilitate treatment involving psychotherapy, aimed at equipping people with personality dysfunction with more personalized adaptive regulation and coping skills to lead more fulfilling lives. (Berk et al., 2018)

The argument that the general neurotic syndrome is not an odd outlier in the diagnostic system but a main component of common mental illness is a powerful one. People with brief episodes of mood disturbance, best identified as adjustment disorders (Chapter 5), attend once or twice only and create few demands on the services. Those with cothymia and the general neurotic syndrome consult repeatedly and, as noted in Chapter 6, are responsible for most of the £7,450 per patient incurred over the first 12 years of the Nottingham Study (Knerer et al., 2005).

So here we are addressing a very important public health issue. In the words of Bernard Lahey (2009), who is using the synonym of 'neuroticism' to describe the general neurotic syndrome, we have a call to action:

> Although not widely appreciated, there is growing evidence that neuroticism is a psychological trait of profound public health significance. Neuroticism is a robust correlate and predictor of many different mental and physical disorders, comorbidity among them, and the frequency of mental and general health service use. Indeed, neuroticism apparently is a predictor of the quality and longevity of our lives. Achieving a full understanding of the nature and origins of neuroticism, and the mechanisms through which neuroticism is linked to mental and physical disorders, should be a top priority for research. Knowing why neuroticism predicts such a wide variety of seemingly diverse outcomes should lead to improved understanding of commonalities among those outcomes and improved strategies for preventing them. (p. 241)

We can safely conclude that the general neurotic syndrome, or any other name that might be chosen for the condition, does indeed add to understanding and cannot be ignored by health services.

8.2 Can the General Neurotic Syndrome Be Assessed Readily in Clinical Practice?

The answer to this question is clearly positive, but it is important to answer it in both primary and secondary care. The two elements of the diagnosis are the presence of cothymia and detection of personality problems mainly, but not entirely, within the domains of negative affectivity and anankastia (we have to get used to these terms). Because the Lewis Prediction almost certainly still applies (i.e., psychiatrists are persuaded by their training to avoid diagnosing anxiety and depression together), it would be best for therapists to provide a self-rating questionnaire such as the Hospital Anxiety and Depression Scale (HADS) to patients seen in their practice.

A large clinical trial carried out over 20 years ago tested whether a clinical guideline combined with education helped general practitioners to diagnose and treat depression more accurately (Thompson et al., 2000). It was ineffective on both counts; a four-hour training session in the active arm of the trial did not improve recognition of depression or the outcome of treatment. The yardstick of accuracy was determined by the score on the HADS – a score of 8 or more on the HADS-D was the index of depression. This was a useful trial to show the limitations of educational programmes in primary care, but what surprised me was the nature of the trial. The fact that the HADS score was kept blind to the participants helped to show that the intervention was unhelpful, but it would have been a much better test to let half of the GP's know the HADS score and the other half be kept blind. Screening for anxiety and depression with the HADS scale is now commonplace in secondary care, most frequently in cancer patients, where it is effective (Mitchell, Meader & Symonds, 2010). If the HADS scale was handed out to patients on their first attendance it could be a useful assessment of cothymia, and a score of 8 or more on the depression scale and 9 or more on the anxiety section, would help to aid the diagnosis. If, within a few minutes of interview, the GP is presented with numerical evidence of both anxiety and depression, the task of detection is almost done. But much more can be done to point out the clinical importance of anxiety combined with depression in primary care. In the ICD-11 classification, there is work being carried out on 28 possible disorders in the primary care version (ICD-11-PHC) (Gask et al., 2018, p. 77) but agreement on these has not yet been reached. One of these diagnoses is 'anxious depression', long argued by David Goldberg (2013) to be an essential element of this classification, and this probably will be included – half a generation after Das-Munshi et al. (2008) pointed out its importance – so it is long overdue.

Eisenberg (1992) wrote a paper 30 years ago that still has relevance today about the ability of general practitioners to identify mental illness and psychosocial problems:

> Goldberg and Gater (1991) have illustrated just how skewed that population sample is. They estimated that one in four of the patients attending a British general practice had one of the common mental disorders: 'becoming anxious, distressed or depressed.' General practitioners recognize only about 40 percent of that group; that is, they identify 1 in 10 of their patients as having psychosocial problems. Of that number, only 20 percent – that is, 2 out of 100 patients – are treated by mental health workers. Yet it is on that unrepresentative subgroup that the official classification scheme has been based. Barrett et al. (1988) examined patients seen in general office practice and found that many of them simply did not fit into the specialists' nomenclature. For one thing, mixed states of depression and anxiety are common. Barrett et al. believe that a purpose-built nosology is needed so that general

medical patients can be sorted out in a fashion useful for making treatment decisions. (Eisenberg, 1992)

I would like to think that matters improved in the subsequent 30 years but as the amount of time that a GP gives to each consultation has steadily reduced – it is now around six minutes – I am not convinced.

It should also be asked, is the diagnosis of general neurotic syndrome of any value to a general practitioner? It is not really a difficult condition to identify but is it really relevant to management. The average GP will know his or her GNS patients only too well; they consult frequently, take up more time than the average consultation, and do not seem to be satisfied with the interventions on offer. When given an opportunity, they will talk at length about every minor symptom and often dominate a clinical interview – reminding me of the Ken Dodd joke: 'I never speak to my mother-in-law; I don't like to interrupt her.'

Bob Kendell has something else to say on this subject:

Many of the conditions which psychiatrists have come to regard as illness, and hence as requiring treatment, do not qualify, or rather there is little evidence at present that they do. The attempt to relieve suffering is medicine's oldest and noblest tradition, and the author is not suggesting that psychiatrists should stop trying to help husbands and wives to live together in harmony, or aimless adolescents to find their feet. But if one is to venture into such areas let it be in full recognition of the fact that in doing so one may be straying outside one's proper boundary, and that in the end it may turn out that other people can deal with such problems as well as or better than the psychiatrist can, and that in these areas their training and their concepts are more appropriate than his. (Kendell, 1975b)

Here I would defend the case that the general neurotic syndrome is a valid area for diagnosis in both primary and secondary care as it such a prominent part of clinical presentation and so cannot be ignored or passed over to somebody else. Later in this chapter the other people who may be able to help more effectively than the GP in dealing with the syndrome are brought on board, but the first stage is to identify the group that needs such additional help.

8.3 Is the Concept of the General Neurotic Syndrome Useful to Patients?

Nobody likes to be called 'neurotic', so the word is normally spoken in the absence of the person to whom it is being applied. Would the 'general neurotic syndrome' be equally unpopular? It might well be, but there is no obvious alternative. What is useful for patients is the introduction of the personality dimension along the lines of: 'It's fairly obvious that you have anxiety/depression/fears or other symptoms, but I think there is something else there as well. I suspect you have personality difficulties that are getting in the way of your recovery. Have I got this wrong?' (Tyrer, 2021). The doctor then introduces the notion of personality problems nagging away in the background and provoking relapse. The results of the Nottingham Study show that the general neurotic syndrome does not go away; in one form or another it stays with you indefinitely. But the important aspect of the syndrome is that it should not handicap a person in the future to the same extent as in the past.

8.4 How Should the General Neurotic Syndrome Be Introduced into Diagnostic and Clinical Practice?

The general neurotic syndrome could be regarded as a synonym for neurosis, but this is not strictly accurate. It is better to think of neurosis as a neurotic spectrum in which the general neurotic syndrome is positioned towards the end of the scale (Figure 8.1).

This condition is seen most often in primary care and it is there that it should be first diagnosed. But GPs are not over-keen on diagnosis in psychiatry, and it is not difficult to see why. As Linda Gask and her colleagues put it:

> Patients in primary care settings are much less likely to present with clearly identifiable diagnostic syndromes. People present with a wide variety of symptoms, concerns, worries, and problems. These are not only undifferentiated as originally described by Balint (1964), but also, crucially, at least at first presentation, unrehearsed by prior discussion with doctors versed in the addenda and language of diagnosis. (Gask et al., 2018, p. 73)

One of the critical words in this passage is 'unrehearsed'. This may not be quite as true today as Dr Google is only too ready to spread diagnoses around like confetti, but it is generally true that in primary care the need for a specific diagnosis is much less important than in secondary care.

But how then can the general neurotic syndrome be identified? It is quite easy. It should be suspected if any of the following apply:

(i) fat-folder patients
(ii) frequent attenders
(iii) failure to respond to standard treatments
(iv) a loquacious mixture of complaints covering many areas of life.

So, within a few minutes of arrival in the surgery the doctor should be able to identify those who may have the general neurotic syndrome. It is fair to add that this is not very different from the way psychiatrists look at diagnosis. Bob found that psychiatrists, both young and old, experienced and inexperienced, made their diagnostic decisions within five minutes of a clinical assessment (Kendell, 1975a). General practitioners probably take only four minutes on a good day.

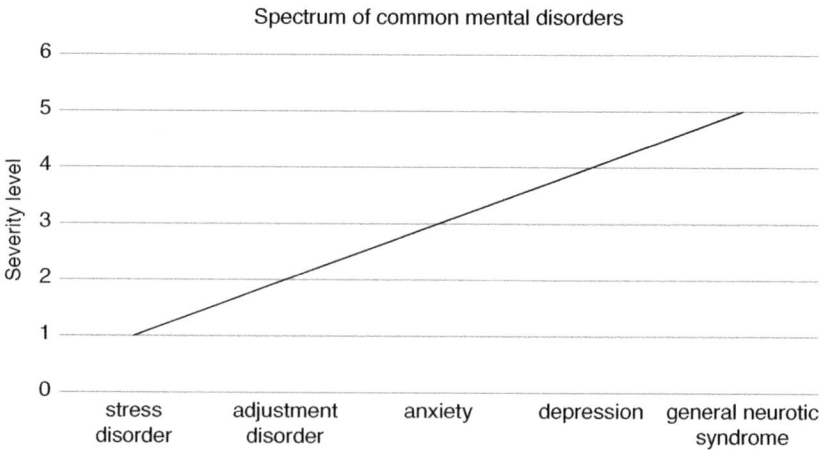

Figure 8.1 The neurotic spectrum of common mental disorders

8.5 How Should the General Neurotic Syndrome Be Treated?

One of the gloomiest views that has been expressed about the Nottingham Study results is along the lines of 'since the results of your study show no benefit from any form of treatment it should only be relegated to the side-lines of care'. Even if that were true, it would not be a reason for disregarding the diagnosis. Randomised trials and large-cohort studies are useful in showing how groups behave but do not identify every outcome. I have misquoted Tennyson in the past in suggesting he might have written a critique about randomised trials: 'so careful of the group they seem, so careless of the single case' (Tyrer, 2008b).

Although the patients with the general neurotic syndrome in the Nottingham Study as a group fared uniformly poorly, a significant number did improve and, at 30 years, 21 of the 46 GNS+ patients were rated as recovered in formal ratings, and all of these had no clinical or social function scores within the range of pathology and had been well for at least two years. These recovered patients were more than offset by the other 25 patients getting worse or staying the same but it is of value to look at why and when the 21 patients recovered during the trial.

This is summarised in Table 8.1. Minor changes have been made to avoid identification of the patients concerned.

Table 8.1 Details of patients rated as recovered at 30-year assessment

Gender	Age at entry (decade)	Initial randomised treatment	Main factors identified as responsible for recovery
M	40–49	CBT	Had mild symptoms at 12 years; had cerebro-vascular accident leading to early retirement from civil service in 1991. Much better mental health from retirement onwards.
F	30–39	CBT	Mental health completely changed when she remarried in 2007. Much happier, spends most of her time with grandchildren who rely on her help greatly.
F	30–39	Diazepam	Very handicapped by anxiety until 2002, which extended to agoraphobia and social anxiety. Better when she moved to village outside Nottingham where she felt less pressured, and also helped greatly by CBT from psychologist.
M	50–59	CBT	A very nervous man with no self-confidence, who after his wife died moved to a village outside Nottingham and was helped greatly in a community retirement scheme that improved his social skills.
F	30–39	Self-help	Two big positive events – happily married in 2001 and moved to West Country in 2006. Keen on self-help and also helping others. Since retirement in 2015 has been involved in much voluntary work.

Table 8.1 (cont.)

Gender	Age at entry (decade)	Initial randomised treatment	Main factors identified as responsible for recovery
F	20–29	CBT	After divorce from aggressive husband in 2001 has been better, especially so after moving to village 20 miles from Nottingham and living alone. 'Happier now than I have ever been.'
M	30–39	Diazepam	Remained on benzodiazepines for many years to combat anxiety symptoms. Moved to Northwest England in 1989. Developed multiple sclerosis (MS) later and had to give up work. Has been better mentally and more accepting of his disability since getting MS.
F	20–29	Self-help	Much better after divorce from husband ten years ago. He was aggressive and blackmailed her by preventing contact with her children. Some help from counselling with psychologist but felt that self-help was the best way forward.
M	40–49	CBT	See full description of patient 86.
F	20–29	Self-help	Much happier since marriage 27 years ago and moving to a new post and home outside Nottingham. On no drug treatment, relies on her own efforts.
M	30–39	CBT	Found working for a major utility very stressful and retired early twelve years ago. Moved to town 15 miles from Nottingham. Worked again but made redundant in 2013. Mental health dramatically improved at that time, loves spare time now and looking after grandchildren.
F	20–29	Self-help	Much better since her divorce in 1989. At that time made visits to GP and out-patient clinics but 'then I noticed I was always much worse after going there so decided to do it all myself'.
F	30–39	CBT	Much better and moved to West Country 10 years ago. New life, new contacts and able to maintain these after husband died. Loves travelling.
M	30–39	CBT	Very much better after stopping work – very physically demanding job – advice to stop drinking and smoking very helpful indeed. After stopping work also learnt to drive, 'one of the best things I ever did'.

Table 8.1 (cont.)

Gender	Age at entry (decade)	Initial randomised treatment	Main factors identified as responsible for recovery
F	20–30	CBT	Much better after leaving Nottingham in 1993 and getting new post in hospital in Birmingham. Very much better. Hardly ever consults doctor. 'I know myself better and now know what to do.'
F	30–40	Placebo	Moved round country in teaching jobs but retired in 2011. Found teaching repetitive and not fully satisfying but after retirement moved to Yorkshire and passed a Master's degree which made her very proud. Brief period on sertraline when depressed but now stopped.
M	20–29	CBT	Much better after moving to Manchester and taking up post in public service. Did well and with pay-out on leaving has set up a construction firm which is very successful.
F	40–49	CBT	Continuously unwell until she separated from her husband and met a new partner – 'completely changed my life'.
F	20–29	Self-help	Better after moving to village 18 miles from Nottingham, but also had persistent phobia of death. Worse after brother and sister died within 5 months of each other 8 years ago but after crisis at this point steadily improved. 'I am coming to terms with the fact that not everybody is the same, that you have to accept things and deal with problems yourself.'
F	20–29	Dothiepin	Moved away to village 8 miles from Nottingham in 1998. Left job in hospital 8 years ago and toured the world for a year. Much better after leaving job and set up beauty clinic from home. Gets nervous at times, but has self-help routines, including mind gym, that keeps symptoms at bay.
M	40–49	CBT	Developed severe attack of meningitis in 1999 which left him with mild memory impairment. But from then on he says he is 'looking after my mental health myself'. Having a severe physical illness has put this in perspective.

NB. The comments in quote marks come from the patients' own comments in filling a section in the interview asking what had helped them most in the study.

The case of patient number 86 in the trial needs a separate description as it describes the biggest change in outcome in any patient in the study. He was recruited to the randomised trial (with panic disorder as well as the general neurotic syndrome). His personality status at entry was at the most severe of all the patients in the study. He was chronically anxious and depressed, was taking large doses of benzodiazepines and antidepressants with very little effect, and was infused with anger about the way he had been treated by his parents, who had always favoured his younger brother, and this anger extended to all members of the family. He continued to be unwell up to the 12-year follow-up point and it looked as though he would have a very poor outcome at 30 years.

He then experienced what could be described as an epiphany moment. At a time when he was feeling more depressed than he had ever done, he took it on himself to walk into a Catholic church in Nottingham. He sat down in one of the pews and a priest came to see him. Our patient professed to no religious faith but found the presence of the priest comforting, and when he left, he was given a rosary. He left the church and made the decision to change his life around. He was going to forget all the past troubles at home and forge a new life for himself. He also resolved to stop all his medication and start afresh with no pharmacological help.

It was a great struggle to get off all his medication, taking nearly two years, but he succeeded. He joined an allotment group, made new friends there who knew nothing about his past, and became highly competent at gardening. At 30 years he could not properly explain what had happened; only that seeing the priest had given him the realisation that he could have a different life. When he was assessed at 30 years, he had symptom scores all below the threshold of pathology and good social function.

Of course, I would love to know exactly what it was that effected the change. In trying to figure this out I think the words of Francis Thompson, himself a lost soul who spent several years homeless on the streets of London, are apposite: When you are at your absolute rock bottom you can sometimes see the way ahead with much greater clarity than ever before, especially if there is a religious connotation.

This is one of the verses from 'In No Strange Land':

> But (when so sad thou canst not sadder)
> Cry;—and upon thy so sore loss
> Shall shine the traffic of Jacob's ladder
> Pitched betwixt Heaven and Charing Cross.
>
> Yea, in the night, my Soul, my daughter,
> Cry,—clinging to Heaven by the hems;
> And lo, Christ walking on the water,
> Not of Gennesareth, but Thames!

Examination of this group of recovered patients throws a new light on the general neurotic syndrome that needs more exposure. Although the group is a heterogeneous one, it is possible to find several common features:

(1) in most cases the improvement followed a very major life event,
(2) a move away from the city of Nottingham was a common feature,
(3) the change induced by the major event was so profound that a complete re-examination of the person's life was initiated,
(4) psychological means of resolving problems were more commonly employed than pharmacological ones.

I should add that our analysis of these issues is still not finalised and will appear in other publications shortly.

These findings point towards a possible way of managing those who present with the general neurotic syndrome. The other findings of the study suggest that this intervention should start early rather than late, as although the patients presented to general practice clinics much earlier than would be expected in an outpatients clinic, nearly a third (32 per cent) had a recurrent disorder on entry to the original trial, and these incurred more costs and a poorer outcome than those who presented with a new episode.

8.6 How Should the General Neurotic Syndrome Be Treated?

Let us start here by returning to the case of Mrs Bennet, who is about to see her physician again. This is the conversation they are now having. Mrs Bennet, as you might expect, is mildly agitated in expectation.

'Mrs Bennet, I have now made a full assessment of your nerves and have come to the following conclusions . . .'

(She interrupts) 'I do hope you can give me good news, doctor, because otherwise I may become quite distraught.'

'As you said earlier Mrs Bennet, you have suffered from your nerves for as long as you can remember. This is an affliction that is likely to continue for quite a long time.'

'Don't say that, doctor. If you cannot offer me hope I am undone. That I cannot tolerate. I can feel another wave coming on. I must lie down.'

'Please let me finish, Mrs Bennet. When I said this is likely to continue for quite a long time this does not mean it has to continue in the same way indefinitely. What you need to do is to organise your life more carefully so that the ups and downs of your nerves can be made tolerable.'

'But how can I do that doctor? Mr Bennet, and my five daughters, lead me up and down with their fancy notions and I cannot keep up with them.'

'You have to adapt Mrs Bennet. You have lived with your five daughters and Mr Bennet for many years and know them, as you said yourself, like the back of your still-elegant hand, if I may so venture a compliment at this difficult time. If you do understand them so perfectly, you should be able to anticipate what they are going to say or do.'

'You flatter me, doctor, but I can see through you. You add compliments to assuage bad news. But when I say I understand them I just mean that I understand they are governed by caprice and impulse. Lydia just needs to see a sergeant from the regiment and she is after him like a moth to a flame. How can I anticipate that?'

'Simply, you need a way of stopping your nerves making an unwanted entrance. You are an intelligent woman and to allow your nerves to dictate is an unnecessary abrogation; they are not worth it. I suggest another experiment. Please write down at the beginning of each day in the next two weeks all the things that are likely to happen on that day and what you can do to avoid your nerves being agitated. There is no need for you to be bullied by your nerves; now is the time to start bullying them in their turn. I am sure if you went through this exercise, you would find an answer. For example, you have told me already that Mr Bennet retires to the library whenever trouble is around. Might it not be possible, Mrs Bennet, for you to retire to the library at these times, just before he plans his escape, and let Mr Bennet deal with any problems that may arise.'

'I am beginning to get an idea what you were talking about, doctor. I think the right word is control. If I can control my circumstances, I can control my nerves.'

'I really think you have it, Mrs Bennet. Up until now you have allowed events in your life to control you; now is the time for you to control them.'

'I don't know how to thank you, doctor. I must go and tell my daughters immediately.'

'I would advise against, Mrs Bennet. You are too ready to confide in others. It leaves you exposed. I think this conversation should remain confidential until I see you again in three months' time. You can tell me then if your nerves have been securely locked away until you permit them an airing.'

This is not an idle sojourn into *Pride and Prejudice*; there is a serious message behind it. The 30-year study of the general neurotic syndrome has established that its symptoms and behaviour will not be changed easily, if at all; that aggressive personal attempts to overcome it are unlikely; and that the best advice in management is to work out a way of adapting to the symptoms and accepting their persistence.

To give you a more apt illustration of ways in which the general neurotic syndrome both progresses and might be treated, I am introducing Lizzie. Lizzie is a remarkably apt equivalent of Elizabeth Bennet in *Pride and Prejudice*, first met on 7th May 1987 when she was 21 and about to enter the Nottingham Study of Neurotic Disorder. She was attending for her first appointment at one of my general practice psychiatric clinics in Nottingham. I do not pretend that I made a full assessment at that time. I was carrying out 19 clinics a month so was very busy, but as I have written elsewhere, it was professionally still the most satisfying part of my career (Tyrer, 2013).

Lizzie has symptoms of both anxiety and depression and a lot of life problems, but the anxiety symptoms predominate, and these are marked at interview. But at this first interview she describes the feelings that hundreds of people are disclosing to doctors and other therapists in clinics every day. These could be lumped together, as I have done in this book, as typical cothymia, but they are not typical; they are unique. Behind these symptoms there is so much more that is normally unsaid and unheard. Now, 34 years later, I have finally opened my ears and eyes and asked for her account in connection with this book and she has responded with eloquence and enthusiasm. I hope her words show this to be far removed from a confession forced on her by my request. In her words, 'it has opened up the lidded boxes of my brain' and she is happy for all to read her account. It is the story of just one of the participants in the Nottingham Study; each of whom could tell much more than was ever disclosed at any interview.

8.7 Lizzie's story

'It is not too difficult to pinpoint when my anxiety crept into my life. Leading up to becoming five years of age, I lived in a much loving extended family, being adored by grandparents, other relatives and, of course, my parents. I may have already picked up on my mother's distress even before then, as she had three children within three and a half years and although she was the most incredible mother, it became clear to those close to her that she was struggling with the demands of home and her own mental health.

Things then changed very quickly for me at such a young age, when unknowing to me, my parents, in an act of kindness, offered board and lodgings to a man who had relocated to the village to take up employment at the local garage. As we were brought up in a very social home, initially I did not feel any fear towards the lodger and in fact I was often told by him 'what a beautiful and clever child' I was.

Obviously, now I realise that he was grooming me, and also my sister who is only thirteen months older than me, but my confident younger brother was too much of a risk to keep silent. Even at the age of three years he had a real sense of self, and he knew nothing about what was happening to his siblings. The insight that I later gained was how vulnerable children can be pinpointed by others to be groomed. By then I also had a baby brother, who would later become the reason why I kept quiet about my sexual abuse as I was told that he would be abused too if I told anyone else about the sexual abuse. Despite hiding in my parents' wardrobe each night before I was told that I had to get into my own bed, there was still no understanding in their minds why I was acting that way. I still have dreams about my parents' wardrobe in which I am hiding Jewish children from Nazis or am telling children to be quiet and hide under the blankets when the family home has been invaded. Once put back into bed, I would surround myself with my cuddly toys as a means of protection, an innocent thought at such an innocent age. I still have those same childhood toys; I cannot part with them as we had a bond which later I realised was a dark secret. The abuse continued to both my sister and me and sometimes it would take place together. By this time, I feared the physical abuse too, with threats of being held against the gas fire if I told anyone. In my mind I think that my abuser was getting worried that he would be found out, but I felt that I had no one to tell. A sense of deep anxiety had already been manifest. I carry this with me today, my dreams are the nightmares of helplessness and of no one listening to me, the frustration of telling the little ones that I was trying to protect not to make a noise or to stay hidden under the covers.

I was already a quiet and sensitive child, but now was I full of fear, inner emotional, and outer physical pain from the sexual abuse inflicted upon me. With no ability of being able to escape from this, I disassociated with drawing, often with messages; if only someone could have paid more attention to the detail within my artwork. There was always a house, with the sun shining above it, but each house never had a front door, I guess that it was my showing there was no escape. Following visits to my doctor for unexplained rectum injuries and the school noticing that my behaviour had become even more withdrawn, the police were alerted and at last we felt able to speak our truth, even though we did not understand what had been happening to us. But I still dreaded going to bed at night or being left alone with this man.

My police questioned my abuser about a theft at the local garage where he worked. I think that at this point I felt able to tell my parents what had been happening as we had to go for a medical examination, but after that time it was never mentioned again, nor did I ever receive professional counselling or an explanation from my parents. The shame intensified and my childhood would be blighted by the preceding year of child sexual abuse; little did I realise then that it would still affect me now. I have PTSD, agoraphobia, depression, chronic anxiety, and a continuing sense of never accepting my achievements in life, still remaining forgotten, misunderstood, and unable to speak about exploitation when it occurs in my adult life.

I have never been a relationship with a man who made me feel that he would protect me. I have no libido and am content to be a single woman; I will not be controlled by a man again. My father was also a controlling man, and I have seen recurring patterns of control in my previous relationships. As an adult, I now need to be independent, self-reliant, and safe. Due to the many fractures I have suffered, leading to lifelong mobility problems, I have not been able to continue with a career that would have got me out of the poverty trap, given me self-worth, and enabled me to mix with like-minded people. But I still want to be independent.

From the moment of my original sexual assaults, I have felt the shame, added to my abuser saying, it was all my fault. The shame was accentuated as I did not have the courage to confide in my parents or be reassured that I had never asked for this to happen. Our family home became dark with secrets, added to by the distress of my parents. We all had to contain this; after all, how had this happened in such a loving and well-functioning family? I could not find the words to write down my emotions, but I could make up poems in my head. My dolls were my friends, they would understand because if I told any of my friends it would be betrayal and more shame and judgement. I still have every toy from my childhood, as each has such significance.

I then learnt to sew, making outfits for my dolls and new soft toys to become part of our protection. I watched my mother sew and then I picked up the basics. My creative world was now full of colour, full of new beginnings as I had produced something that I could relate to, and give to someone else (this being new outfits for my dolls). Throughout junior school, we were told about road safety and how a policeman would be coming to school each year to talk to us. Every day, I had this feeling of dread, could this be the day that I am pointed out to the school as that bad girl who had done bad things! This is a burden that no young child should have to carry. I did not realise that I was the victim of the most horrific abuse, because it was not spoken about again at home, as my parents thought that it was better to sweep it under the carpet and once again contain it.

As I reached adolescence, the words of my abuser were still being repeated in my mind, that because I was a pretty child he could not help himself. I did not wear makeup, once my breasts had started to develop, I strapped them down, I did not tell my parents that I had started my periods. My anxiety and fear that I would get noticed by older men made me miss out on the adventures of teenage years. I excelled at school, but we did not have the career advisors at school that I believe might have led me to a rewarding career in the arts!

Yet I would be allowed to change my bedroom and redecorate, and I would make my own soft furnishings. Our home was always filled with our school friends and my mother would make us all beautiful meals in which all of us would help.

When my mother died, I was just seventeen years of age. It was as though the world had stopped again. We had just been on two wonderful family holidays, and I was beginning to feel that I could now feel safe to go to discos and become a teenager. Everything at my home changed again, its darkness and distress filled every part of our home. There we were, four traumatised teenagers with a father who did not know how to cope. My sister had a place at a university in London and my youngest brother was about to go to secondary school. My role in becoming a mother to everyone became more intense, as I was working full time and my father had teaching commitments in the evenings as well.

My mother was loved but vulnerable. She had the ability to make everyone feel that they were special and important. So, I naturally took the children who were bullied at school home for tea; that was my way of trying to save them. I also knew that my mother could not cope with running the house, so I would do the housework before my father came home so that he would not shout at us or see that my mother was not functioning. I took on my mother's emotional pain; we often heard her crying, she suffered from agoraphobia, and self-harmed which she always said were accidents. I just wanted my father to be calm and my mother to be happy. In many ways she was like a child; we had to fetch our own school uniforms, wash our own clothes, and organise ourselves to function at school without the other children knowing how difficult it was for us. Again, we were sweeping it all under the carpet.

I worried about my mother, and noticed that I was unable to sleep. I paced around, as if I laid down in bed everything would be so much worse in my thoughts, with an overwhelming feeling of despair and grief. This had happened when I studied for my exams, but also, I realised as a consequence of my previous abuse, I did not really sleep when I went to bed. I lay there pretending to be asleep, praying that the bedroom door would not open so that my sister and I would not be taken out of our bunk beds. I had the same recurring dream for many years, a nightmare of being rolled down a hill in a wooden barrel and if your number was called you had to go down the hill once again, even if you had the fear that your barrel would break. I feared that I would become like my mother, who, due to her own mental illness, never realised what an impact her behaviour had on our childhood. This included arguments with my father, whom she felt was still a 'mummy's boy', holidays ruined by my mother crying each morning in bed, seeing her biting her fingers down to the bone when stressed, showing the distress felt throughout the home of an unhappy marriage accompanied by her own feelings of failure.

Hope came when I started a job with Laura Ashley. I was surrounded by colours each day – fabrics, wallpaper, beautiful clothes. My career took off at an early age and by eighteen I was put forward for management posts, helping to train staff and open new branches throughout the country. My training notes were used in the company staff manuals. Each day at work gave me an escape. I could immerse myself in creativity and, more importantly, become financially independent. But pressure grew at work and I felt guilty about being away from my father and two younger brothers. But my career escalated very quickly, perhaps too quickly, and I felt that I may have been promoted too soon.

I had the ability to do the job and was very successful in my management role. But the long hours, lack of support at work, combined with uncertainly about where my next management role would be in the UK, added to my anxiety. The pressure began to affect me. I started to experience agoraphobia and dissociation again. I felt I had too many responsibilities too young, and I regretted not being able to socialise with friends of my own age.

After several years, I started suffering more severe symptoms of depression and anxiety. I felt dissociated and unable to cope, I become paranoid that I was failing and developed the 'imposter syndrome' that I had from primary school, feeling that whenever I did well, I was not being the real person inside. This was when I suffered my first nervous breakdown. I still dream about my time at Laura Ashley, at least once a fortnight, but these dreams are distressing as I never get paid or acknowledged in them, no matter how much I try to be back as part of the team on the shop floor in Nottingham. I know now that I should have stayed there for much longer and not taken up a management post only a year after my mother's passing. It was a very strict work environment and very regimented. I have spoken to others who worked alongside me and each said the same.

Further education provided me with a sense of fulfilment. I passed each exam with distinction and went on to take exams at the highest level offered on each course. Money was very tight, but I supported myself through bar jobs. At this time, I went into rented accommodation in the form of bedsits. I felt however that I was living the student years that I never had. It didn't include drinking alcohol or one-night stands, more that I was helping myself to achieve better work prospects and prove to my family that I wasn't such a failure!

My empowerment is creativity, the ability to make items from fabric, yarn, a paint brush, cookery, and floristry, just to name of few of skills that I have learnt mainly with the help of

YouTube as many creative courses are no longer available due to lack of funding. These classes gave me structure, a reason to get up and meet like-minded people, and make many long-term friends. I found that many other people who attended the classes were not working because of anxiety and depression. We all shared how anxious we were when going to the courses initially, but then we found creative expression, a feeling of self-worth, simply just belonging and feeling understood.

But my life has taken many unexpected and tragic turns and prevented normal employment. I was away enjoying a family holiday in the UK when I fell some distance and broke my left ankle and heel bone. I was told at the age of thirty-three years that I probably would not walk with ease again, but my strong coping mechanisms made me believe otherwise. Despite being put into non-weight-bearing plaster for much of the next fourteen years, I never lost sight of gaining back my independence and my determination not to have to depend on anyone else. Unfortunately, the bone density was reduced in my right kneecap, right wrist and my right foot and ankle, and it needed many operations before I was able to walk again.

It was decided that I should go back to stay with my father for several weeks following each stay in hospital. Spending time back at our family home was of much comfort but also full of traumatic memories. I coped by sewing using my left hand. I listened to talking books and took my mind off an uncertain future by making my brain remember all the happy times from my childhood, being surrounded by my siblings, cousins coming to stay and the thoughts of love and understanding for my beloved mother. It was a healing time for me and my father; we spoke in depth about how both of our lives had challenges but being part of a supportive and loving family always got us through. Having long-lasting mobility issues combined with chronic anxiety has reinforced the difficulties of living off very little income and the battles to be rehoused in social housing suiting my needs. The housing shortage means that you have long waiting lists and little option of which area you will be rehoused.

I still have a constant fear of being exploited as throughout my life I have been seen as a soft touch, and so have been taken advantage of by people who appear to be your good friends and neighbours. I have always lived alone and, due to my medical issues, I tend to feel very isolated which in turn makes me feel very vulnerable. For some reason, I still trust the word of others; my life experiences have not made me cynical. I still want to protect those who struggle too, almost as if they were the lost child that I once was, internally begging for support.

I had my crafts to fill my days whilst recuperating, getting joy and fulfilment in completing items that I gave to others. Although my right wrist still has not got full movement and flexibility, I learnt how to sew and crochet. I got out an old paint set and produced paintings of my friend's pets. I had not painted since I was at school and yet the gift was still there. I amazed people around me with my talents, some of which had lain dormant, but I was pleased I still had artistic flair. My work has inspired others to heal themselves through creativity, gain self-confidence through producing items, joining groups to meet new friends. My sense of pride came back as I was reinforced and could no longer ignore the reactions of other people who saw my work. I found that my obsessionality and need for perfection lessened as there are no rules to follow if you have your own ways of expressing yourself.

I remember that I told my psychiatrist once, that I just wanted to be 'ordinary', to be able to do a 9–5 life like others around me who went to work but did very little outside of that, and I got a reply that has always stayed with me, 'you will never be ordinary, Lizzie, as you were born to be extraordinary!'

Lizzie finishes her account with the comment: 'I wish all can understand the creativity that has helped me to find peace, fulfilment, and purpose.'

There are many insights into neurosis that come from this frank account, part harrowing, part sympathy-provoking, and part fortifying. Some might even think that this is the best way to formulate the subject; a book of 210 life accounts like Lizzie's might offer more than the selective groupings of what are no more than collective episodes of events and outcomes. But there are elements of Lizzie's story that help to understand the findings of the Nottingham Study and also reinforce them.

8.7.1 Sexual Abuse

Lizzie may or may not have been of an anxious disposition when she was very young but there is absolutely no doubt that the sexual abuse added to it immensely. Although we did not formally assess sexual abuse as part of the Nottingham Study, the main assessor in the latter stages, my wife, Helen, worked in a genitourinary medicine department, where abuse is always asked about as a matter of course. A history of physical or sexual abuse was present in approximately a quarter of all cases in our study.

Lizzie, sadly, describes a very typical account of the consequences of child sexual abuse. Becoming withdrawn and getting anxious; not being able to disclose; taking refuge in toys, painting and writing, are all common response to this uttermost violation of intimacy. What might have been done to help Lizzie at this point and would it have prevented all her future symptoms? This is impossible to answer, but we have clues that awareness is moving in the right direction, and if she had a sympathetic counsellor who could assist in showing that no blame whatsoever could be attached to her, that there was no reason for shame, and that her self-worth could be preserved, how might have her life have changed for the better. If the right combination of disclosure, support, enrichment, and prevention could be implemented everywhere, it would have a major effect on the long-term outcome of so much of mental illness. It is worth noting in the Nottingham Study that those who presented with recurrent symptomatology generally had a worse outcome than those who presented with new symptoms, so it could be argued that any intervention for those with early trauma who presented in adult life was already too late.

8.7.2 Family Dynamics

One of the elements scored in the scale for the diagnosis of the general neurotic syndrome is the presence of a similar condition in a first-degree relative. This is an acknowledgement to both the genetic contribution to the disorder (Hettema et al., 2001) and the behavioural effects of modelling described in Section 1.2 point 4. Children are very sensitive to parental behaviour – this is shown very well in Lizzie's account – and may imitate facets of this in their own development.

8.7.3 Employment

Despite this early adversity, including the death of her mother, Lizzie was able to gain useful employment. Then she made the decision to give her job up at Laura Ashley in favour of further education. This almost certainly was a mistake. She had shop-floor and management skills and was successful, and if she had received the right level of support and advice at this point everything might have turned out very differently. As it was, her financial future from then onwards became very insecure. This was aggravated intensely by the injuries she had received it to her foot, which under normal circumstances would have been expected to lead to full recovery. This was not achieved and I suspect her care and surgical interventions could have been improved.

8.7.4 Psychological Treatment

Lizzie also received several sessions of private psychotherapy as well as psychotherapy support from a highly regarded consultant psychotherapist. But the psychotherapist felt at the point he saw Lizzie she was too disorganised to 'use more productively more intensive explorative work or other forms of challenging psychotherapy'. We cannot presume the exact nature of these sessions, carried out at a critical time in Lizzie's life, but it could be argued that this was an opportunity missed.

8.7.5 Suicidal Behaviour

'Is there any point to which you would wish to draw my attention?'
'To the curious incident of the dog in the night-time.'
'The dog did nothing in the night-time.'
'That was the curious incident,' remarked Sherlock Holmes.

This is the famous passage from *Silver Blaze*, the short story by Arthur Conan Doyle, 1892. The curious incident that should attract our attention in Lizzie's life is the complete absence of both suicidal thinking (found in our repeated assessments over 30 years) and suicidal behaviour in her story. This might be thought to be unusual, not least as such behaviour is described as a very frequent consequence, some claim a uniform one, of sexual abuse and its 'borderline' sequelae. But because no element of suicidality was shown, despite massive mental suffering, it deserves analysis. We have several clues in Lizzie's story. She never lost hope, she maintained optimism in adversity, and, perhaps most importantly, her creative juices were always active. What her creativity and optimism illustrate were her personality strengths. When these are lacking, suicidal behaviour is more common (see Table 7.10) but because Lizzie had elements of all five of the personality strengths identified in Chapter 7 – forcefulness, emotional toughness, cautiousness, independence, and discernment – she never became completely overwhelmed by the disasters that surrounded her.

In this respect, we can see common elements in Lizzie and Jane Austen's Mrs Bennet. Both showed determination and strength in their core beliefs; both stood up to a great deal of strain, especially within the family; both had a long-term strategy that was never lost; and, in both cases, their persistence to follow their dreams was not idle fantasy, but a constant awareness that others could be brought on board and, in time, support them.

So here we find some positive aspects of the term 'neurosis'. The people who show these features in their personal and medical interactions are not weaklings who creep about under the strong legs of others. They, often as a consequence of adversity, have inner toughness that may need to be harnessed in therapy.

Because we have generally ignored the nature of Galenic syndromes like the general neurotic syndrome, we are almost starting from scratch in determining a way forward. But we have clues. If the findings of the Nottingham Study are confirmed in other populations, it will be necessary for NICE (National Institute of Health and Care Excellence) and other bodies to provide guidance for the management of cothymia and associated personality disturbance.

I end this book by prematurely giving some advice to NICE in this task, in which I will return to the new definition of neurosis in its rightful place as a Galenic syndrome. In so doing, I will use the clumsy but cleverly ambiguous text common to NICE documents that is always necessary when there are elements of uncertainty:

(1) People with neurosis should never be excluded from services or dismissed as untreatable.

(2) It is necessary to provide autonomy and choice, working in partnership with those who have neurosis, taking account of their own preferences in treatment, and allowing them to make their own decisions about managing their condition, which may be a long-term one.

(3) Develop an optimistic and trusting relationship with those with neurosis, exploring all their personality strengths in addition to helping with immediate symptoms.

(4) Always bear in mind when providing services for neurosis that many people will have experienced deprivation, rejection, abuse, and trauma in the past, and while their experiences are sometimes the butt of jocular amusement, casual dismissal, or passive acceptance, these people have been subject to considerable suffering and should always be respected.

(5) Community mental health services should carry out a full review of all patients with neurosis at least annually, examining what progress has been made and what new interventions might be needed and implemented.

(6) Long-term psychotropic medication should be reviewed carefully as there is little evidence that it provides continuing benefit, but nonetheless accept that a minority of patients may give cogent reasons for its value.

(7) Attention should always be paid to changes in life style and environmental adjustments as many people with neurosis may experience positive change when placed in different settings or altering their life priorities. This discussion should always be carried out in a collaborative fashion with any decisions to change being supported and embraced fully by the person concerned, not forced externally by a therapist.

I could add more here but it might be indulging too much in speculation. Still, I like to think that if Mrs Bennet was presented with this advice today, not only she but the Lizzies of this world, would all be pleased. They might all choose to go off in entirely different directions if the treatment known as Adaptive and Acceptance Therapy (AAT) (Tyrer, 2021, pp. 97–99) was developed in a personal way. Adaptive and Acceptance Therapy is an extension of nidotherapy, a collaborative treatment in which the patient makes the major decisions with the help of the therapist and which has at its theme, 'find content in the environment'. (The aim is to find the best possible adaptation of the personality to the setting). Once this has been achieved, or even if it has failed and the best environment has not been found, the process of acceptance takes place and the person is asked to look at the advantages of what at first appears to be an unattractive position.

So in Lizzie's and in Mrs Bennet's case we are not offering anything approaching a cure or even a major resolution of their symptoms. Lizzie is now settled with a clear path ahead but will continue to need some support. As for Mrs Bennet, one hopes that with two of her daughters settled in matrimony with two husbands 'in possession of a small fortune' she might be more satisfied with the results of her endeavours. But of course, she will not be until the future of Longbourn is assured, and she still has three rather silly daughters yet to develop skills to enter early nineteenth-century society. By improving the balance in the household between Mr Bennet and herself, she could make some progress, and in time could develop a space for herself to carry out what she would like to do, indulging in herself rather than perpetually worrying about what others are doing or not doing.

She need not be a candle blowing in the wind, instead, an established matriarch with others admiring her ability to act as a marriage broker, even though such a title may be partly undeserved. She is a resourceful woman and I have no doubt she could persuade one of her daughters and a husband to come to live in Longbourn and deflect the odious Mr Collins from his intention to purchase the property. She could retire to separate quarters and appear from time to time to deliver her nuggets of advice to those who are still prepared to hear. And I am sure she would make an excellent grandmother as she is so good at telling stories. She might even create one about her own life, showing that for some the possession of neurosis can be a proud exemplar of success.

Appendix
Personality Assessment Schedule
(Tyrer & Alexander, 1979)

(Bona fide researchers can use this instrument without the need for formal permission, but are advised to test it out for agreement first in order to understand its scope and scoring range.)

Personality Assessment Schedule (PAS) – Original version (Tyrer & Alexander, 1979)

This schedule is designed to formalise the assessment of personality disorder and may be used with any subject irrespective of psychiatric status. The way in which the schedule is used will depend on the current mental state of the patient and an assessment of this is a necessary precursor to the personality ratings. It is recommended that the screening schedule of the Present State Examination or SCID (Structured Clinical interview for DSM-III) be used for the mental state examination, but, if this is not possible, sufficient information should be obtained from the history and examination to make a diagnostic formulation of any psychiatric problems, which should be recorded on the assessment form. If this is not carried out, there is a danger that the personality ratings will be contaminated by the mental state.

There are 24 personality variables to be assessed in the schedule. Each of these can be rated by interview with the subject or interview with an informant.

An interview with an informant is desirable in all cases. The interview with the subject is not necessary if he or she is unable to give coherent answers to questions because of gross abnormalities in mental state; the interview with the informant indicates that there has been a marked qualitative change in the subject's personality so that replies to questions about past personality are unlikely to be correct; or the subject displays severe memory disturbance, whether of organic or psychological origin, and is unable to recall aspects of his or her premorbid state. If an interview with an informant is not possible, additional independent information about personality may be obtained from other sources (e.g., general practitioner, social worker, probation officer), if this information is considered valid. If several informants are available, the final score can be a composite of those in which the most reliable informant carried the greatest weight.

Use of the Schedule

(1) The initial questions for each personality variable are obligatory. The questions preceded by an asterisk are amplifying questions which may be asked in response to the subject's initial reply. The questions in brackets are direct closed questions which may be asked if replies to other questions have been evasive, contradictory, or vague. Although the questions are confined to a specific personality variable, there is sometimes overlap with other variables. It may therefore be necessary to re-rate the variable later in the interview.

(2) Ratings of severity: The ratings are made on a nine-point scale for all variables. The number is recorded in the appropriate box at the side of each item or an accompanying sheet. The scale is specifically designed to record abnormal personality traits and most normal variation will occur between scores 0 and 3. The greater the severity of the trait, the greater will be the rating. In addition to the specific points mentioned for each scale, the following general principles should be used to determine the score for a particular trait. (The word trait is synonymous with personality variable in this account, although it is less often used for severe personality disturbance).

0   Trait absent. Presence of the trait is undetected both in respect of feelings and of behaviour.

1   Subject recognises the presence of the trait but it is shown chiefly in terms of feelings rather than behaviour. When the trait does affect behaviour, it is not a habitual response so much as a tendency to indulge more in that type of behaviour when several choices are open. Knowledge of how the subject spends spare time may help with this rating, as it is in spare-time activities that the element of choice is most obviously shown. (An informant is unlikely to make a distinction between 0 and 1 ratings.)

2   Personality trait is definitely present and affects behaviour, but only to a limited extent. It is not associated with problems in occupational, social, and interpersonal life. The changes in behaviour produced by the trait are such that those close to the subject will notice them but most friends and acquaintances would not.

3   The personality trait markedly affects feelings and behaviour. The presence of the trait may be noticed by others who are not closely related to the subject and may occasionally give rise to the problems in occupational, social, and interpersonal life. However, these problems will seldom be persistent and those around the subject can normally accommodate to them without much difficulty.

4   The personality trait is marked and is apparent to the subject and to most people who have frequent contact with the subject. The trait produces some difficulties in occupational, social, and interpersonal adjustment and this tends to be of a mild but persistent nature.

5   The personality trait is marked to both the subject and most people who come into contact with the subject. It has a marked influence on behaviour and leads to problems in occupational, social, and interpersonal relationships. This rating differs from 4 in that the problems lead to more serious difficulties in adjustment in society and marked underachievement (e.g., inability to settle in one job, refusal to meet people, episodic aggression).

6   Personality trait has a major influence on behaviour and tends to affect all aspects of life. The problems in occupational, social, and interpersonal relationships are such that major breakdown occurs (e.g., divorce, social isolation, prolonged unemployment), as a direct result of the personality abnormality.

7   The personality trait is so marked that it is noticed by almost all who come in contact with the subject, even those who only see the subject once. Independent life in the community is impossible because of the severity in occupational, social, and interpersonal relationships so some form of supervision or continuous support is necessary.

8 The personality trait dominates behaviour completely (therefore it cannot be given to more than one rating in the schedule). The disturbance produced by the trait is so marked that prolonged periods of institutional care (e.g., hospital, prison, nursing home) take up a large part of the subject's life history in the absence of any formal illness.

Note: most normal variation is accounted for between the ratings of 0 and 3. Only a small number of individuals rate higher scores than 3. The key issues in deciding whether a score of more than 3 is justified are as follows:

(a) The production of problems in daily living because of the severity of the trait.
(b) The suffering and underachievement that the trait produces.
(c) The inability of those around the subject to deal with these problems without asking for additional (often professional) help.

An informant's information is primarily of value for ratings of 3 and upwards. A reliable subject is best fitted to rate lower ratings as these have little or no persistent effect on behaviour.

In all instances of abnormal personality traits, try and get the subject or informant to provide examples of the problems produced by the trait.

Assess the reliability of the subjects' and informants' replies at the end of the interview and score on the nine-point scale. Wherever the informants' and subjects' ratings for an item differ by three or more points, ask further questions and, where possible, obtain independent information about the trait in question.

Additional Notes on PAS
Procedure for Scoring

It will be noticed on the final scoring sheet there is a space for 'the final score'. If the reliability of the informant's ratings is considered to be greater than or equal to the subject's ratings, the final score will normally consist of the informant's ratings alone. If, however, the difference between informant's and subject's ratings for a personality attribute is greater than two points, it is advisable to ask further questions to establish the reasons for the discrepancy, possibly with both informant and subject present together. On an individual item it may also be considered that the subject's ratings are more reliable than those of the informant even though the rest of the ratings may be more accurately determined by the informant. In such instances the scoring may more closely approximate to the subject's ratings for that item.

If the subject's ratings are to be considered more reliable than those of the informant (which is particularly likely if the informant is not a close relative and has only known the subject for a limited period), the subject's ratings will take greater precedence in the final scoring. However, any informant rating that is greater than 3 must be carefully followed up by further questioning if it significantly disagrees with that of the subject. This is because any abnormal behaviour as a consequence of the personality attribute is likely to be more accurately detected by the informant than by the subject.

If the informant is not available, the subject's ratings alone can be used although this is much less satisfactory than having the informant's ratings also. If the subject's ratings are to be used, as much independent information as possible about premorbid personality is needed to corroborate the subject's ratings. This may be possible from past medical or social records but recording of major life events (see Useful Facts, p. 143) may be useful.

This is administered before the PAS, preferably with other independent information as well, and any relevant positive findings introduced at the appropriate point in the PAS when this is administered subsequently. The subject will then have to explain the reasons for the apparently abnormal behaviour and, if the abnormality is judged to be related to a personality attribute, it will be scored appropriately. The additional schedule therefore serves in some way as a lie schedule.

When scoring each rating, use the notes below each personality trait for guidance only. The scoring should follow the principles outlined in the Use of Schedule section pages 133 and 134 for all traits.

Comparison of Scores in Different Subgroups of Patients

The individual scores for personality attributes can be compared separately by the usual statistical methods.

Useful Facts

Sometimes both subjects and informants have a distorted impression of previous personality and make it sound more favourable than it really was. The rater therefore needs as much information as possible about the patient's past experience so that this can be introduced into the questioning at relevant points in the interview. Here follows a list of some of the important events that are frequently affected by personality characteristics. The rater should have information about these events, preferably obtained independently, before the interview. If this is not possible, questions should be put to both subject and informant during the interview. It would be wrong to assume that any of these events are necessarily associated with personality abnormality but they are useful anchor points around which questions about personality can be asked. If there are serious discrepancies between independent evidence of these events and the subject's or informant's responses, the rater should resolve these before making a final score for that personality item. As in other parts of the schedule, independently derived information is given greater weight when making this decision.

(1) *Marital relationship.* If unmarried, has the subject ever cohabited? If married or divorced, how many times have the couple separated for any reason during marriage?
(2) *Child care.* Have there been any problems with the children of the patient? Have any children been involved with the police or official agencies and have they ever been in care?
(3) *Has the subject ever been in debt.* What were the circumstances?
(4) *Employment.* How many jobs has the subject had since leaving school? What were the circumstances of leaving these jobs? Was the subject ever sacked from a job or did they leave because of problems with colleagues?
(5) *Legal.* Has the subject ever been convicted of an offence? If so, what was the offence and outcome?
(6) *Alcohol.* Does the subject drink, take illegal drugs, or gamble? If so, have any problems arisen as a consequence of these activities?
(7) *Housing.* How many addresses has the subject had in the last 10 years? What were the reasons for moving? Has the subject ever been homeless?
(8) *Adolescent problems.* Did the subject have any problems when attending school after the age of 11? If so, what was the outcome?

Interview Procedure

It is helpful to have a checklist of ratings of severity for each personality trait and the aforementioned eight-point Useful Facts section when interviewing the patient or informant. These are appended and may be detached for ease of reference when interviewing. The list of facts may be completed after the interview if necessary.

Subject

I am going to ask you some questions about the type of person you are normally.

*I am trying to find out what you were like before your present problems began.

In answering these questions, I would therefore like you to think about your personality as it has been throughout your life. I am going to ask you some more questions about this but first of all how would you describe your personality in a few words? (Note main features and record on sheet at end of schedule).

Informant

I am going to ask you some questions about the type of person S is normally.

*I am trying to find out what S was like before his/her present problems began.

In answering these questions, I would therefore like you to think about S's personality as it has been throughout his/her life. I am going to ask you some more questions about this but first of all how would you describe S's personality in a few words? (Note main features and record on sheet at end of schedule).

1 Pessimism

Subject

Do you get depressed easily or are you reasonably cheerful?
Are you pessimistic or optimistic about the future or do you just take it as it comes?

(1)

*Have you always felt depressed and low spirited, or has this only happened recently?
*Do other people notice it? (Give examples)

(Has this affected you at work, at home and with friends? In what way?)
(Have you ever thought seriously about suicide?)

Further questions may be needed to separate episodes of depressive illness from persistent depressive attitudes and behaviour.

Informant

Does S get depressed easily or is he/she reasonably cheerful?

Is he/she pessimistic or optimistic about the future or does he/she just take it as it comes?

☐ (2)

*Has S always felt depressed and low spirited or has this only happened recently?
*Does S appear gloomy to other people?

(Has this affected him/her at work, at home and with friends? In what way?)
(Do people avoid S because he/she is so miserable?)

Subject/Informant

Note	Ratings 1–3	A pessimistic outlook on life with no effect on behaviour.
	Ratings 4–6	Depressive behaviour including social withdrawal and morbid depression to the extent that others notice and are affected by the behaviour.
	Ratings 7–8	Persistent pessimism and depressive behaviour with almost complete withdrawal and isolation.

Ratings of 5 and above are only justified when depressive feelings and behaviour, associated with hopelessness about the future, are present or have been present in the absence of formal psychiatric illness. Do not include recurrent depressive illness in this category unless the personality between episodes is also abnormal or there is evidence that S has been clinically depressed all his/her life. Short periods of pessimism or depressed feelings of less than two weeks should be regarded as evidence of lability of mood rather than evidence of abnormal pessimism. If in doubt, delay rating until lability trait scored.

2 Worthlessness
Subject

How do you think of yourself in relation to other people? Do you feel better, worse, or about the same?

☐ (3)

*Do you feel inferior to others? In what way? For how long?
*How does it affect you?

(Have you always felt like this or only just recently?)

*Do you think your like would have been different if you did not feel inferior to others? In what way?

(Do you feel useless or worthless most of the time?)
(Have you ever thought you deserved more out of life?)
(How would you feel if you were promoted at work?)

Informant

How does S think of himself/herself in relation to other people?
Does he/she feel better, worse, or about the same?

☐ (4)

*Does he/she feel inferior to others?
*Do others notice this?

(Has he/she always felt like this or only just recently?)

*Does he/she think his/her life would have been different if he/she did not feel inferior to others? In what way?

(Does S feel useless or worthless most of the time?)

Subject/Informant

Note	Ratings 1–3	Mild feelings of inferiority, fully compensated and not obviously apparent to others.
	Ratings 4–6	Strong feelings of inferiority, affecting behaviour. Subject will not do things he/she is capable of because of abnormally low self-esteem. At least some impairment at work and social adjustment.
	Ratings 7–8	Strong feelings of inferiority amounting to worthlessness. Because of those feelings subject requires continuous reassurance and support. Not able to work regularly or make any useful relationship.

Do not confuse worthlessness with depression although the two often coexist.

3 Optimism

Subject

I asked earlier whether you were normally a cheerful person. (Refer to answer)

☐ (5)

*Are you more or less cheerful than most other people?
Have you always felt very cheerful no matter what has been happening in your life?

*Sometimes cheerfulness and overconfidence can lead to difficulties in life, such as over-spending or making plans to do something which cannot succeed. Is this true of you?
*Would you describe yourself as too optimistic? (Examples of problems associated with optimism.)

*Have you any special abilities that make you feel optimistic and successful?

(Have you ever been in debt or got into trouble in any way because of overconfidence?)

Exclude problems associated with irresponsibility or childishness.

Informant

I asked earlier whether S was normally a cheerful person. Do you think of S as cheerful? Would others describe him/her as cheerful? Has S always felt very cheerful no matter what has been happening in his/her life?

☐

☐ (6)

*Sometimes even cheerfulness can lead to difficulties in life, such as overspending or making plans to do something which cannot succeed.
*Would you describe S as too optimistic? (Examples of problems associated with optimism.)

*Does S think of himself/herself as a special person who is bound to succeed?
(Has S ever been in debt or got into trouble in any way because of overconfidence?)

Subject/Informant

Note	Ratings 1–3	Subject is more cheerful than most others and is capable of communicating his/her cheerfulness to them.
	Ratings 4–6	Over-cheerfulness leads to unrealistic ambitions and aspirations, including overspending, overconfidence and impaired judgement, so subject may be sacked from work or be in serious debt. Subject remains optimistic and self-important in spite of these problems.
	Ratings 7–8	Breakdown in relationships, inability to maintain stability in any aspect of social, occupational, or interpersonal life because of abnormal cheerfulness, over-optimism and self-importance.

To merit a high rating, the optimism has to be more or less continuous and not part of the manic phase of manic-depressive illness. Short periods of abnormal optimism of less than two weeks should be regarded as evidence of lability of mood rather than evidence of abnormal optimism. If in doubt, delay rating till lability trait is scored.

4 Lability
Subject

Do your spirits}   change from day to day or week to week, or do they/does it remain
Does your mood}   more or less the same?

☐

☐ (7)

*Are these changes connected with what is going on in your life or are they separate?

*How long do they last?
*Do they lead to problems?
(Can you predict your changes in mood?)
(How often do you laugh or cry?)

Informant

Does S's mood change from day to day or week to week, or does it remain more or less the same?

☐

☐ (8)

*Are these changes connected with what is going on in his/her life or are they independent?
*How long do they last?
*Do other people notice these changes? Do they lead to problems?

(Is S unpredictable because of these sudden changes in mood?)
(How often does he/she laugh and cry?)
(Do you ever feel that he/she can turn these feelings on when he/she wants?)

Subject/Informant

Note Ratings 1–3 A tendency towards mild exaggeration of mood swings in response to life changes.

Ratings 4–6 Marked lability, noticeable to others and leading to problems because of strength of mood swings. Most mood changes responsive to life events but may be independent. Unpredictability of subject's behaviour because of mood change also a source of difficulties.

Ratings 7–8 Breakdown in social, occupational, and personal relationship because of abnormal swings in mood. In these instances, it would be more likely that the changes are independent of life events so that they cannot be manipulated in any way. What is known as 'cyclothymia' will be included here if the swings in mood occur at least as frequently as once every two weeks. If they occur less frequently than this, but still produce important personality problems, then the relevant rating should be included under the pessimism and optimism scales.

5 Anxiousness
Subject

Are you normally an anxious or a calm person?
When things go wrong in your life (e.g., illness in family, accident) do you get more nervous, the same, or less nervous than most people?

☐

☐ (9)

*Do you ever worry about things that most people would not be concerned about?
(Give examples)
*Do you show your nervousness to other people or do you cover it up?
*Have you always been an anxious person?

(Do you worry about something or someone most of the time?)
(Has your anxiety ever led to problems?) (Specify)

Informant

Is S normally an anxious or calm person?
When things go wrong in his/her life (e.g., illness in family, accident) does he/she get more nervous, the same, or less nervous than most people?

□ (10)

*Does S ever worry about things that most people would not be concerned about?
(Give examples)
*Do other people notice that S is an anxious person or does he/she keep it to himself/herself?
*How has this worrying affected S?

(Does S worry about something or someone most of the time?)

Subject/Informant

Note	Ratings 1–3	Mild anxiety-proneness which is normally suppressed so that others are not aware of it.
	Ratings 4–6	Anxiety noticeable to others, leading to changes in behaviour.
	Ratings 7–8	Frequent or continuous free-floating anxiety of such severity that breakdown in social adjustment occurs.

Life-long phobic anxiety may contribute to this rating but the severity of the rating would depend on the same categories mentioned in the outline to scoring (i.e., it is the extent to which it interferes with personal and social adjustment that determines the rating).

6 Suspiciousness
Subject

How well, in general, do you get on with other people?
Do you normally trust them or are you suspicious of them, at least at first?
How long does it take for you to get to know people before you will trust them?

□ (11)

*Do you tend to worry about what is going on behind your back?
*Do you ever think that other people might be against you or criticise you unfairly?

(Have you many friends?)
(Are you worried in case someone might find out what you have been saying to me?)

Informant

How well, in general, does S get on with other people?
Does S normally trust them or is he/she suspicious of them, at least at first?
How long does it take for him/her to get to know people before he/she will trust them?

[ ] (12)

* Would you say that S is a suspicious person?
* Does he/she have many friends? (If no) Is this because he/she will not trust anybody?
*Is S a jealous person?

Subject/Informant

Note	Ratings 1–3	Mild feelings of suspiciousness, not noticed by others. Subject tends to have relatively few friends but is capable of close relationships and will trust those he/she knows well.
	Ratings 4–6	Problems in social adjustment because of abnormal suspiciousness. Takes a very long time to get to know people and only trusts a very small number of people. Feels that others criticise him/her without adequate cause.
	Ratings 7–8	Breakdown in relationships and social adjustment because of abnormal suspiciousness. At extreme ratings, the patient is completely isolated because he/she feels all are against him/her.

7 Introspection
Subject

Do you think a great deal about how you feel and what you do or do you think about them very little?
Do you prefer being on your own to being with other people?

[ ] (13)

*Are you a person who spends a lot of time thinking? (If yes) What about?
*Are you an introvert?
*Are you like this all the time or only when there is a problem on your mind?

Informant

Does S think a great deal about how he/she feels and what he/she does or does he/she think about them very little?

Does S prefer being alone to being with other people?

☐ (14)

*Is S an introvert?
*Is S completely bound up in himself/herself? How often?
*Does S appear to live in a world of his/her own?
*How does this affect his/her relationship with other people?
*Do other people notice that S is like this?

Subject/Informant

Note	Ratings 1–3	Mild introspection and introversion, not noticeable to others.
	Ratings 4–6	Problems in adjustment because of excessive rumination and introspection, often with a tendency to indulge in fantasy. These feelings may lead to problems by indecision, impaired judgement, and poor relationships.
	Ratings 7–8	Completely bound up in self to the exclusion of other matters, indulges in much fantasy. Self-neglect frequent.

8 Shyness
Subject

Are you normally a shy person or are you confident with other people?
Do you get to know people quickly or do you take a long time before feeling at ease with them?
Do you lack self-confidence?

☐ (15)

*Do you ever go out of your way to avoid people because of shyness?
*Do you have difficulty in making friends because you are shy?
*Would you like to feel more at ease with people? Has shyness caused problems for you?

(Do you feel uncomfortable even in the presence of friends?)
(Are you feeling shy or uncomfortable now?)

Informant

Does S get to know people quickly or does he/she take a long time before feeling at ease with them?
Is S normally a shy person or does he/she have no difficulty getting on with people?

Is S a self-confident person?

(16)

*Does he/she ever go out of his/her way to avoid people because of shyness?
*Does S have difficulty in making friends because S is shy?
*Do other people notice that S is shy?
*Has shyness caused problems for S?

(Does S feel uncomfortable even in the presence of friends?)

Subject/Informant

Note	Ratings 1–3	Mild shyness, but this is compensated and others do not notice it.
	Ratings 4–6	Excessive shyness and lack of self-confidence leading to avoidance of people and personal discomfort when with people.
	Ratings 7–8	Subject unable to work adequately or make relationships because of symptoms. In severe cases may be completely isolated.

It is important to exclude natural aloofness and detachment from shyness – the former group are not distressed in the company of other people; shyness is always associated with some feelings of anxiety.

9 Aloofness
Subject

Are you a person who likes to stay apart from other people or do you like to have close relationships?

Have you any really close relationships? (If no, does this bother you?)   (17)

Do you need people in any way or can you do without them?
(Would you mind living entirely on your own without any contact with other people?)
(Do others ever say you are stand-offish or aloof?)

Informant

Is S an isolated/aloof person who likes to stay apart from other people or does he/she like to have close relationships?
Has he/she any really close relationships?

(18)

*Does S ever appear stand-offish or detached to other people?
*Is S happier when he/she is on his/her own?

(Do other people tend to stay apart from S?)
(Has this tendency to be aloof led to any problems in S's life?)

Subject/Informant

Note	Ratings 1–3	Mild detachment leading to a reluctance to be involved in close relationships. Not noticeable to others, and adequate relationships made with close friends and relatives.
	Ratings 4–6	Abnormal aloofness noticeable to others and leading to problems in social adjustment, mainly in interpersonal relationships.
	Ratings 7–8	Excessive detachment and lack of interest in other people. No close relationships. Indifference to other people's feelings and opinions.

Lack of interest in other people is unrelated to shyness or psychiatric symptomatology such as social fears. Subject does not feel distressed with other people and merely has no interest in them.

10 Sensitivity
Subject

Are you a {touchy/sensitive} person or does it take a lot to upset you?
How do you react to criticism? (Give examples)

(19)

*Do people ever say you are too touchy?
*How long does it take for you to get over criticism?

(Have any of my questions upset or disturbed you in any way?)
(Do you tend to take things personally?)

Informant

Is S a {touchy/sensitive} person or does it take a lot to upset him/her?
How does S react to criticism? (Give examples)

(20)

*Have people got to be careful what they say to S in order not to upset him/her?
*Do people ever say S is too touchy?
*Does he/she take a long time to get over criticism?

(Has this sensitivity led to problems in S's relationships with others?)

Subject/Informant

Note   Ratings 1–3   Mild sensitivity. May be upset easily but does not show it except to close friends and relatives.

Ratings 4–6   Excessive personal sensitivity with a tendency to self-reference (e.g., feels people are being critical when they are not). This leads to problems in social adjustment (e.g., frequent changes of job, broken relationships).

Ratings 7–8   Excessive sensitivity leads to breakdown in social performance. Extreme tendency to self-reference.

Sensitivity to the feelings of others is not an abnormal phenomenon and should not be included in this rating. This rating is concerned with personal sensitivity and touchiness. If in doubt about this rating, delay till ratings of vulnerability and irritability are made. Also differentiate between sensitivity and suspiciousness. Although the two may overlap, sensitivity leads to emotional distress whereas suspiciousness is usually independent and may frequently be prominent in insensitive people.

11 Vulnerability
Subject

Do you find that when things go wrong in your life it disturbs you a great deal or do you remain on an even keel?
Does it take you a short time or a long time to get back to normal after some mishap (e.g., illness in family, accident, loss of job)?

(21)

(How do you think you would cope with a crisis such as death in the family, car accident or loss of your job?)

Informant

Does S find that when things go wrong in his/her life it disturbs him/her a great deal or does he/she remain on an even keel?
Does it take S a short time or a long time to get back to normal after some mishap (e.g., illness in the family, accident, loss of job)?

(22)

*Does S need to be protected from unpleasant things because others know he/she will take them very badly? (If yes) Could you give an example?
*Are other people aware that S is vulnerable? How do they show it?

(Do you protect S from unpleasant events?)

Subject/Informant

Note	Ratings 1–3	Reacts more than most to adversity but does not show these feelings to others.
	Ratings 4–6	Abnormally vulnerable, reacts excessively to adversity, so leading to social maladjustment for a prolonged period. Eventually, however, more normal functioning is resumed until the next adverse episode.
	Ratings 7–8	Subject vulnerable to even the minor stresses of life to which he/she reacts as though they were major problems. Breakdown in social adjustment because of this.

It is important to separate vulnerability from sensitivity and resourcelessness. Although all three may be present in one individual, the characteristics are separate. The sensitive person is touchy and reacts easily to implied criticism, the vulnerable person reacts to major life events by feelings of distress which may take a long time to resolve and are not commonly associated with compensatory action, and the resourceless person reacts to adversity by not coping and just giving up. When assessing vulnerability, do not include sensitivity and resourcelessness.

12 Irritability
Subject

Are you an irritable or a placid person?
Are you impatient at times? Under what kind of circumstances?
How do you show it?

(23)

*Do you keep it to yourself or do other people notice that you are impatient and irritable?
*Does this lead to problems in your relationships with other people?

(When was the last time you were really irritable?)
(How did you show this?)

Informant

Is S an irritable or a placid person?
Is he/she impatient at times? Under what kind of circumstances?

How does he/she show it?

(24)

*Does he/she keep it to himself/herself or do other people notice that S is impatient and irritable?
*Does this lead to problems in S's relationships with other people? (Specify)

Subject/Informant

Note	Ratings 1–3	Mild irritability, kept under control.
	Ratings 4–6	Abnormally irritable. Leading to social adjustment problems (e.g., poor relationships with others).
	Ratings 7–8	Severe irritability, making it very difficult for subject to make adequate relationships with others. Inability of the subject to cope in any environment which involves sudden changes because of severe irritability.

In making this rating, impulsiveness and aggression should be excluded. An impulsive act is followed by regret. Irritability is largely shown in verbal responses and does not include physical violence, which should be scored under aggression. 'Passive-aggressive' features may be included here if the irritability leads to procrastination, obstruction, and delay in completing tasks.

13 Impulsiveness
Subject

Do you always think carefully before you do something or do you act on impulse?

(25)

*Have you ever done things on impulse and regretted them afterwards? (Give examples)
*Have to ever been in trouble because you are impulsive? (Give examples)
*When you have been impulsive has it ever harmed other people?

If the 'Useful Facts' section (p. 143) suggests impulsivity is a problem (e.g., criminal offences), mention them here if subject answers negatively.

Informant

Does S think carefully before he/she does something or does he/she act on impulse?

(26)

*Does he/she ever do things on impulse and regret it afterwards?
*Has S ever been in trouble because he/she is impulsive? (Give examples)
*Has his/her impulsiveness ever harmed other people?

(Has S had problems with drugs or drink because he/she is impulsive?)

Subject/Informant

Note	Ratings 1–3	Mild impulsiveness, not noticeable to others, causing no problems in social adjustment.
	Ratings 4–6	Impulsiveness associated with regret which has led to problems of social adjustment (e.g., loss of job).
	Ratings 7–8	Frequent impulsiveness leading to criminal behaviour and/or breakdown in social functioning throughout adult life.

As impulsiveness may sometimes be associated with aggression, this rating may be delayed until aggression is assessed.

14 Aggression
Subject

Do you lose your temper easily or does it take a lot to make you angry?
When you get angry how do you show it?

(27)

*Have you ever lost control completely?
*Are you normally like this or only on certain occasions (e.g., after heavy drinking)?

(Do you ever react by physical violence?)
(Have you ever been in trouble with the law?)

Informant

Does S get angry easily or is he/she generally placid?
When S does get angry how does he/she show it?

(28)

* Has he/she ever lost control completely?
* Is he/she normally like this or only on certain occasions (e.g., after heavy drinking)?
* How do other people react to S's violence? What problems does it cause?

(Does he/she ever react by physical violence or does he/she keep it to himself/herself?)
(Has S ever been in trouble with police/law?)

Subject/Informant

Note	Ratings 1–3	Anger and aggression felt frequently but kept to himself/herself.
	Ratings 4–6	Aggression abnormal and leads to social difficulties (e.g., trouble with police), and violence at home. Do not rate criminal offences here unless they are a direct consequence of aggressiveness.
	Ratings 7–8	Breakdown of social adjustment with long history of antisocial behaviour, usually with criminal record.

15 Callousness
Subject

Are you easily affected by other people's feelings or can you ignore them?

(29)

* Do you care much about other people? (Do you care at all?)

(Do you find it difficult to sympathise with and understand other people's feelings?)
(Have you ever enjoyed hurting other people?)

Informant

Is S easily affected by other people's feelings or can S ignore them?

(30)

*Does S care much about other people?

Does S find it difficult to sympathise with and understand other people's feelings?

*Does he/she ever appear to get pleasure from hurting people in any way?

*How does this affect his/her relationships with other people?

(Has he/she ever hurt people (physically or mentally) deliberately?)
(Give examples)
(Is S callous or sadistic?)

Subject/Informant

Note	Ratings 1–3	Mild insensitivity and indifference to others feelings.
	Ratings 4–6	Cold and indifferent to the extent that S is only capable of a few relationships, and these are rarely close.
	Ratings 7–8	Marked callousness with or without sadistic behaviour, leading to breakdown in social functioning and frequent criminal involvement.

16 Irresponsibility
Subject

Do you ever do things without caring about the consequences or are you always careful in what you do?
Would you describe yourself as a responsible or an irresponsible person?

(31)

Do you ever get into serious difficulties because of irresponsibility (e.g., into debt, criminal acts, sexual difficulties)? How has irresponsibility affected your life? (Give examples). Bring up any information derived from the section 'Useful facts' if negative answers given but past history suggests irresponsibility.

Informant

Does S ever do things without caring about the consequences or is S always careful in what he/she does?
Would you describe S as a responsible or an irresponsible person?

(32)

*Does he/she ever get into serious difficulties because of irresponsibility (e.g., into debt, criminal acts, sexual difficulties)?
*How does this affect his/her relationships with others? How has irresponsibility affected his/her life? Has it caused serious problems?

Subject/Informant

Note	Ratings 1–3	Mildly irresponsible, feelings kept under control, not noticed by others or, if manifest, not causing real problems.
	Ratings 4–6	Highly irresponsible, takes risks repeatedly, problems in social adjustment (e.g., in debt, frequent accidents, unwanted pregnancies). Do not rate criminal offences automatically unless they stem from irresponsibility.
	Ratings 7–8	Irresponsibility so great that S needs to be constantly supervised and cannot live independently because of this.

17 Childishness
Subject

Do you ever act in a childish way or would you regard yourself as fairly mature?
Do you ever manipulate people to get your own way?

(33)

*Do you like being the centre of attention?
*Have you ever acted selfishly, only thinking of yourself?
(Has this led to problems?)

Informant

Does S ever act in childish ways or would you regard him/her as fairly mature?
Does he/she ever manipulate people to get his/her own way?
Has this ever led to problems?

☐ (34)

*Is S a selfish person who only cares about himself/herself?
*Does he/she appear to be younger than his/her years?
*Does he/she like being the centre of attention?

(How does this affect his/her relationships with others?)
(Has he/she any mature relationships?)
(Do other people tend to treat S as a child?)

Subject/Informant

Note	Ratings 1–3	Self-centred attitudes with occasional childish behaviour but this is seldom noticeable to others.
	Ratings 4–6	Immature behaviour and marked selfishness leading to social adjustment problems.
	Ratings 7–8	Severe childishness, cannot live independently because of this. All relationships involve others supervising or caring for S.

18 Resourcelessness
Subject

When you are faced with a challenge do you usually respond to it well or do you give in to it?
When there are problems in your life do you usually tackle them alone?
Are you somebody who can normally solve your own problems?

☐ (35)

*How have you coped with major problems in the past? (Get examples)

(When was the last time you coped with a serious problem on your own?)

Informant

When S is faced with a challenge does he/she usually respond to it well or does he/she give in to it?

When there are problems in S's life does he/she usually tackle them alone or does he/she need help from others?

[ ] (36)

*Does S constantly need support to cope with life's problems?
*How does this affect his/her relationships with others?
*How has S coped with major problems in the past?

Subject/Informant

Note	Ratings 1–3	Copes with problems with some difficulty but does not involve others to an unnecessary extent.
	Ratings 4–6	Others involved in coping with S's problems, impairing social functioning. Frequent problems in work.
	Ratings 7–8	Unable to cope with life's practical difficulties without continuous support. Not able to live independently because of this.

19 Dependence
Subject

Do you rely on other people a great deal or are you an independent person?

[ ] (37)

*Do you find it difficult to make up your mind without involving others?
*How would you like to live and/or work alone?

(Who do you depend on most?) (In what way?)
(Would you like to be less dependent?)
(Has your dependence led to problems in your relationships?)

Informant

Does S rely on other people a great deal or is he/she usually independent?

[ ] (38)

*Does he/she find it difficult to make up his/her mind without involving others?
*Do you think S could cope with living and/or working alone? What would happen?

(Do you think S is too dependent? On whom?)
(Does this lead to problems?) (Give examples)
(Has he/she always been like this?)

Subject/Informant

Note | Ratings 1–3 | Some dependence in excessive need for advice and reassurance from close relatives or friends but behaviour seldom abnormal.

Ratings 4–6 | Excessive reliance on others, leading to social adjustment problems.

Ratings 7–8 | Completely dependent on individual group or institution. Unable to work or function independently at any level.

20   Submissiveness
Subject

Do you give in easily to others or do you stand up for yourself?

(39)

*Do you go along with decisions made by others even if you feel it is the wrong decision?
*Do you prefer to avoid arguments?
*Do people ever take advantage of you? (Give examples)

(Are you easily dominated?)
(Do you wish you could stand up for yourself better?)

Informant

Does S give in easily to others or does he/she stand up for himself/herself?

(40)

*Does S go along with decisions made by others even if he/she feels they are the wrong decisions?
*How does this affect relationships with others?
*Do people ever take advantage of S because they know he/she will not retaliate?

(Is S easily dominated?)
(Is he/she afraid to say what he/she really thinks?)

Subject/Informant

Note | Ratings 1–3 | Mild submissiveness and compliance, but stands firm on major issues.

Ratings 4–6 | Very submissive, unwilling to express own views, is dominated in most relationships.

Ratings 7–8 | Gives in to everybody, no independent function, exploited by others. Breakdown in social functioning.

21 Conscientiousness
Subject

Are you normally a fussy or a carefree person?
Do you plan everything down to the last detail or do you seldom plan anything in life?

(41)

*Do people ever say you are too fussy or conscientious, or even a perfectionist?
*Do you wish you were less conscientious?
*Are you a person with high standards?
*Does conscientiousness ever lead to problems in your life? (Specify)

(Did you worry that you might be late today?)
(If I had been late, would it have upset your routine?)
(Do you think you work harder than the average person?)

Informant

Is S normally a fussy or a carefree person?
Does he/she plan everything down to the last detail or does he/she seldom plan anything in life?

(42)

*Do people ever say S is too fussy or conscientious, or even a perfectionist?
*How does this affect his/her relationships with others?
*Is he/she a person with high standards?

Subject/Informant

Note	Ratings 1–3	Over-fussy and conscientious, preoccupied with routine and excessively meticulous, but no social adjustment problems.
	Ratings 4–6	Abnormal conscientiousness, plans excessively far ahead, adjustment problems because of need for meticulous planning.
	Ratings 7–8	Excessive conscientiousness accompanied by doubt. Unable to achieve anything as the smallest of tasks becomes a major enterprise. Unable to work or use leisure time, leads to interpersonal breakdown. In severe cases subject will usually have many obsessional symptoms.

In making a rating do not include obsessional symptoms (i.e., symptoms which the subject recognises to be silly and consciously tries to overcome), unless these are part of the underlying personality of the subject. Also recognise that conscientiousness is thought to be a favourable personality trait and may be exaggerated by S or informant.

22 Rigidity
Subject

Do you find difficulty in adjusting to new situations or are you an adaptable person?
Do you get upset if your plans are changed for any reason or are you flexible?

(43)

*Can you adjust to others who act or feel differently from you (e.g., at work, with family)?

(Do you always have to have your own way?)

Informant

Does S find difficulty in adjusting to new situations or is he/she an adaptable person?
Does he/she get upset if his/her plans are changed for any reason or are they flexible?

(44)

*Can he/she adjust to others who act or feel differently from him/her (e.g., at work, with family)?
*Is he/she a person of fixed ideas?
*Do other people get upset with S because he/she is inflexible?
(Give examples of problems caused by inflexibility.)

Subject/Informant

Note	Ratings 1–3	Rigidity present but attempted compensation by subject leads to no social adjustment problems.
	Ratings 4–6	Rigidity extreme, refuses to change, often dominating others. Marked problems in social adjustment because of rigidity, although if subject is driving and energetic, he/she may appear successful initially.
	Ratings 7–8	Inflexibility so severe that life is completely ritualistic and impairment of adjustment so marked that independent life is impossible.

23 Eccentricity
Subject

Do you think you are very different from other people? In what way?

(45)

*Have you any unusual habits or interests? What are they?
*Have you any unusual beliefs in things like telepathy and mind control?

(Have these beliefs caused problems in your life?)

(Direct questions may be asked about any eccentric features noted at interview.)

Informant

Do others ever regard S as eccentric in any way? In what way?

(46)

*Has he/she any unusual habits or interests? What are they?
*Does he/she tend to conform with other people or is he/she unaware of them?
*Does he/she deliberately set out to shock people by being unconventional?
*Has he/she any unusual beliefs about telepathy and mind control?
(Do you find his/her thoughts and speech difficult to follow?)
(Can you give examples and problems they have caused?)

Subject/Informant

Note	Ratings 1–3	Mild eccentricity, often deliberately stressed because it does not conform, but no social adjustment problems.
	Ratings 4–6	Marked eccentricity. S unable or unwilling to conform, recognised as odd by others, marked social impairment. Has odd thinking, speech, and beliefs that cause problems in adjustment.
	Ratings 7–8	Behaviour and attitudes so bizarre that life in society impossible without supervision.

A low rating should be given if the subject acts in an eccentric way to attract attention. The true eccentric is oblivious to others' reactions. Any unusual beliefs or perceptions may only be rated if they are independent of mental illness such as schizophrenia.

24 Hypochondriasis
Subject

Do you worry a great deal about your health or do you seldom give it a thought?

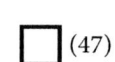 (47)

*When you have been ill, have you worried that it might be more severe than it turned out to be?
*Are you more concerned about your health than most other people?

(How often do you visit the doctor? What for?)
(Have you ever been really well?)

Informant

Does S worry a great deal about his/her health or does he/she seldom give it a thought?

☐ (48)

*When he/she has been ill, has he/she worried it might be more severe than it turned out to be?
*Is S more concerned about his/her health than most other people?
*Do you or other people think of S as a hypochondriac?

Subject/Informant

Note	Ratings 1–3	Mild hypochondriasis. Over-concerned about minor illness and health (e.g., takes vitamins or health foods regularly).
	Ratings 4–6	Hypochondriasis marked. S frequently considers himself/herself to be ill even when physically healthy. Social adjustment problems; hypochondriasis affects behaviour and relationships.
	Ratings 7–8	Hypochondriasis dominates S's life. Considers himself/herself to be ill despite contrary evidence. Unable to live independently because fears about health dominate behaviour.

Many people with a history of mental illness are naturally concerned about its likely recurrence and its effects on other people. Do not rate such concern as abnormal unless it is excessive.

Reliability of subject

On the basis of your interview, do you consider the subject to have been a reliable witness?

Note	Rating 0	Highly reliable witness. Evidence from behaviour and demeanour at interview and any previous knowledge of witness all consistent.
	Ratings 1–3	Probably a reliable witness but independent information lacking.
	Ratings 4–6	Possibly an unreliable witness from demeanour at interview but no independent evidence of this.
	Ratings 7–8	Unreliable witness. Report inconsistent with previous knowledge of witness and evidence of incorrect report from demeanour at interview.

☐ (49)

Reliability of informant

On the basis of your interview, do you consider the informant to have been a reliable witness?

Note	Rating 0	Highly reliable witness. Evidence from behaviour and demeanour at interview and any previous knowledge of witness all consistent.
	Ratings 1–3	Probably a reliable witness but independent information lacking.
	Ratings 4–6	Possibly an unreliable witness from demeanour at interview but no independent evidence of this.
	Ratings 7–8	Unreliable witness. Report inconsistent with previous knowledge of witness and evidence of incorrect report from demeanour at interview.

☐ (50)

Combining Subject and Informant Information

The following procedure is used when both subject and informant versions are available and the assessor wishes to combine them:

(i) If both informant and subject receive the same ratings the combined score is the same;

(ii) If the informant scores differ from the subject scores on one or more ratings decide the 'most accurate' score based on (a) item being tested (e.g., aggression towards others more likely to be rated better by informant, wish to be solitary more likely to be rated better by subject), (b) level of severity: scores of 4 or higher more likely to be rated accurately by the informant, low scores of 2 or less more likely to be rated accurately by subject (since expression of trait not always shown in general behaviour);

(iii) If more than one informant has completed scores, combine informant ratings in a similar way but ensure that more credence is given to assessments that (a) include knowledge of subject in premorbid (i.e., before mental state diagnosis) state, (b) are dispassionate and independent of personal animosity towards the subject, (c) are based on contact with the subject in a range of situations, not just one (e.g., workplace).

Personality Assessment Schedule – Scoresheet

Name:		Date:		Rater:		
			Write rating 0–8 in appropriate box			
Variable	No.	Box no. Sub.		Box no. Inf.		Final score
Pessimism	1	1		2		
Worthlessness	2	3		4		
Optimism	3	5		6		

(cont.)

Variable	No.	Box no. Sub.	Box no. Inf.	Final score
		Write rating 0-8 in appropriate box		
Lability	4	7	8	
Anxiousness	5	9	10	
Suspiciousness	6	11	12	
Introspection	7	13	14	
Shyness	8	15	16	
Aloofness	9	17	18	
Sensitivity	10	19	20	
Vulnerability	11	21	22	
Irritability	12	23	24	
Impulsiveness	13	25	26	
Aggression	14	27	28	
Callousness	15	29	30	
Irresponsibility	16	31	32	
Childishness	17	33	34	
Resourcelessness	18	35	36	
Dependence	19	37	38	
Submissiveness	20	39	40	
Conscientiousness	21	41	42	
Rigidity	22	43	44	
Eccentricity	23	45	46	
Hypochondriasis	24	47	48	
Reliability of information		49	50	

(Name: Date: Rater:)

COMMENTS (Problems in scoring to be noted here) . . . .
. . . .

Revised Scoring of Personality Disorder Using PAS (with ICD-10 and DSM-IV Updates)

The schedule is scored in the usual way and a final score decided for each personality variable before embarking on classification.

Stage 1

Examine all 24 scores. If none is greater than 2, code as 'normal personality' and do not proceed further.

Stage 2
Compute scores for individual personality groupings as follows:

(1) *Sociopathic* – add together the scores for variables 12, 13, 14, 15, and 16, divide total by 5 and subtract from this the sum of scores for variables 2, 21, and 23 divided by 30.

(2) *Passive-dependent* – add together the scores for variables 5, 11, 17, 18, and 19, divide total by 5 and subtract from this the sum of scores for variables 15, 22, and 23 divided by 30.

(3) *Anankastic* – add together the scores for variables 7, 10, 21, 22, and 24, divide total by 5 and subtract from this the sum of scores for variables 13, 15, and 16 divided by 30.

(4) *Schizoid* – add together the scores for variables 6, 7, 8, 9, and 23, divide total by 5 and subtract from this the sum of scores for variables 4, 12, 14, divided by 30.

(5) *Explosive* – add together the scores for variables 12, 13, 14, and 16, divide total by 4 and subtract from this the sum of scores for variables 2, 8, 20, and 21, divided by 40.

(6) *Sensitive-aggressive* – add together the scores for variables 6, 10, 12, and 14, divide total by 4 and subtract from this the sum of scores for variables 3, 23, and 24, divided by 30.

(7) *Histrionic* – add together the scores for variables 4, 11, 17, and 19, divide total by 4 and subtract from this the sum of scores for variables 9, 15, 22, and 23 divided by 40.

(8) *Asthenic* – add together the scores for variables 5, 10, 18, and 20, divide total by 4 and subtract from this the sum of scores for variables 3, 14, and 15 divided by 30.

(9) *Anxious* – add together the scores for variables 5, 8, 20, and 21, divide total by 4 and subtract from this the sum of scores for variables 3, 14, and 15 divided by 30.

(10) *Paranoid* – add together the scores for variables 5, 6, 10, and 11, divide total by 4 and subtract from this the sum of scores for variables 2, 15, and 23 divided by 30.

(11) *Hypochondriacal* – add together the scores for variables 5, 19, 21, and 24, divide total by 4 and subtract from this the sum of scores for variables 3, 16, 20, and 23 divided by 40.

(12) *Dysthymic* – add together the scores for variables 2, 8, 9, and 21, divide total by 4 and subtract from this the sum of scores for variables 3 and 14 divided by 20.

(13) *Avoidant* – add together the scores for variables 5, 7, 8, and 11, divide total by 4 and subtract from this the sum of scores for variables 10, 12, 14, and 23 divided by 40.

Rating of Severity of Personality Disturbance
The 'adjusted' score for each of the 13 personality types is used. For the first four types (sociopathic, passive-dependent, anankastic, and schizoid), a score of 2.5 or more indicates simple (mild) personality disorder, and a score of 2–2.49 indicates personality difficulty. For the remaining nine personality types (explosive, sensitive-aggressive, histrionic, asthenic, anxious, paranoid, hypochondriacal, dysthymic, and avoidant), a score of 2.75 or more indicates personality disorder, and 2.25–2.74 indicates personality difficulties. When a score in one cluster (sociopathic, passive-dependent, anankastic, or schizoid) only is 3.75 or greater, the personality disturbance is also classed as personality disorder. When a score of 2.75 or greater is found in more than one cluster, the personality disturbance is classified as complex (moderate) personality disorder unless there is a mean difference of 1.0 or greater between the highest score in one cluster and the highest score in any of the remaining ones. (This reflects the overlap between traits, when very high scores can affect several clusters.)

Severe Personality Disorder

This is decided by a two-stage process. A score of 4.0 or more for one of the flamboyant cluster personalities (sociopathic, sensitive-aggressive) together with a score of 3.0 in one of the other personality disorders (except histrionic) suggests severe personality disorder. In the second stage, the assessor has to decide the following:

(i) Does the personality disorder create significant distress and dysfunction not only to immediate friends, family, or household members but also to wider society (defined as all other people apart from friends, household, and family members)?

(ii) Is the extent of such distress great enough to affect at least 50 other individuals apart from family members and close friends as a direct consequence of the personality disorder (e.g., people alter the times of arriving and leaving their houses in order to avoid encountering the individual)?

(iii) Is there clear evidence that threat is created by the pattern of personality characteristics in that fear of mental or physical harm is an intrinsic part of the distress or discomfiture created by the personality abnormality (e.g., fear of unprovoked violence)?

If the answers to all these questions are positive, the individual can be described as having severe personality disorder.

In obtaining this information, it is important to use more than one source, as individuals with these disorders are unlikely to admit all these negative characteristics readily or spontaneously. It is also important for the assessor to make their own judgement as to whether the fears and concerns of the individuals concerned are justified and not based on stigma or prejudice.

Combining Diagnoses

In some studies, it may be necessary to combine the diagnoses to obtain numbers large enough for analysis. This can be done by reducing the numbers of personality types to four – antisocial, dependent, inhibited, and withdrawn.

These are combined according to the following scheme.

Sociopathic	
Explosive	Antisocial group
Sensitive-aggressive	
Passive-dependent	
Histrionic	
Asthenic	Dependent group
Anankastic	
Anxious	
Hypochondriacal	Inhibited group
Dysthymic	
Schizoid	
Paranoid	Withdrawn group
Avoidant	

Key Traits

For some studies, research workers prefer to use a dimensional assessment of personality rather than a categorical one. This has the advantage that all subjects being tested with the schedule will have a key trait score for each of the main personality groups and this may be useful in studies that are looking at personality traits and characteristics rather than specific personality disorder. The key traits score for each of the four major personality types is calculated as follows:

(1) *Sociopathic* – add scores for variables 12, 13, 14, 15, and 16, and divide total by 5.
(2) *Passive-dependent* – add scores for variables 5, 11, 17, 18, and 19, and divide total by 5.
(3) *Anankastic* – add scores for variables 7, 10, 21, 22, and 24, and divide total by 5.
(4) *Schizoid* – add scores for variables 6, 7, 8, 9. and 23, and divide total by 5.

The nine subcategories of personality disorder can also have their key traits scores calculated in a similar way. However, it should be noted that many of these overlap as they are subcategories of the main ones and therefore their key traits scores will be similar. Explosive (impulsive) and sensitive-aggressive personalities are subtypes of the sociopathic group; histrionic and asthenic personalities are subtypes of the passive-dependent group; anxious, hypochondriacal, and dysthymic personalities are subtypes of the anankastic group; and paranoid and avoidant personalities are subtypes of the schizoid group.

(4) *Explosive (impulsive)* – add together the scores for variables 12, 13, 14, and 16, and divide total by 4.
(5) *Sensitive aggressive* – add together the scores for variables 6, 10, 12, and 14 and divide total by 4.
(6) *Histrionic* – add together the scores for variables 4, 11, 17, and 19, and divide total by 4.
(7) *Asthenic* – add together the scores for variables 5, 10, 18, and 20, and divide total by 4.
(8) *Anxious* – add together the scores for variables 5, 8, 20, and 21, and divide total by 4.
(9) *Paranoid* – add together the scores for variables 5, 6, 10, and 11, and divide total by 4.
(10) *Hypochondriacal* – add together the scores for variables 5, 19, 21, and 24, and divide total by 4.
(11) *Dysthymic* – add together the scores for variables 2, 8, 9, and 21, and divide total by 4.
(12) *Avoidant* – add together the scores for variables 5, 7, 8, and 11, and divide total by 4.

Personality Assessment Schedule: DSM-IV Version

Although the PAS was developed before DSM-III was introduced and includes some items that are not present in DSM personality disorders (e.g., hypochondriasis), there is still a considerable degree of overlap between the personalities derived from the PAS and those in DSM-IV. The scoring system below is suitable for reaching a DSM-IV diagnosis with the PAS. This is a simple procedure that can be done by hand as well as using a short computer program.

Add the ratings for each of the four variables and divide by four to get the mean score. A mean score of 2.75 or greater indicates a DSM personality disorder. Simultaneous presence of several personality disorders is permitted in DSM-IV, but the personality type with the highest score could be regarded as the most serious.

DSM-IV coding	Personality type	
301.00	Paranoid	suspiciousness + sensitivity + vulnerability + irritability (6+10+11+12)
301.2	Schizoid	introspection + aloofness + eccentricity + pessimism (7+9+23+1)
301.22	Schizotypal	shyness + eccentricity + suspiciousness + aloofness (8+23+6+9)
301.5	Histrionic	lability + dependence + childishness + irresponsibility (4+19+17+16)
301.7	Antisocial	callousness + aggression + impulsiveness + irresponsibility (15+14+13+16)
301.8	Borderline	lability + impulsiveness + aggression + worthlessness (4+13+14+2)
301.82	Avoidant	vulnerability + shyness + anxiousness + submissiveness (11+8+5+20)
301.6	Dependent	dependence + submissiveness + resourcelessness + sensitivity (19+20+18+10)
301.4	Obsessive-compulsive	conscientiousness + rigidity + introspection + anxiousness (21+22+7+5)
301.81	Narcissistic	childishness + vulnerability + optimism + irritability (17+11+3+12)

ICD-10

ICD-10 personality disorders show a close relationship with the PAS sub-classification. The following diagnoses can be regarded as equivalent:

Sociopathic	(PAS)	and	Dissocial	(ICD-10)
Passive-dependent	(PAS)	and	Dependent	(ICD-10)
Explosive	(PAS)	and	Impulsive	(ICD-10)
Sensitive-aggressive	(PAS)	and	Dissocial	(ICD-10)
Histrionic	(PAS)	and	Histrionic	(ICD-10)
Asthenic	(PAS)	and	Dependent	(ICD-10)
Avoidant	(PAS)	and	Anxious	(ICD-10)
Schizoid	(PAS)	and	Schizoid	(ICD-10)
Paranoid	(PAS)	and	Paranoid	(ICD-10)
Anankastic	(PAS)	and	Anankastic	(ICD-10)

Other diagnoses in the PAS can be categorised under 'Personality Disorder – other' in ICD-10.

References

ABC-H Investigators, Roush, G. C., Fagard, R. H. et al. (2014). Prognostic impact from clinic, daytime, and night-time systolic blood pressure in nine cohorts of 13,844 patients with hypertension. *Journal of Hypertension, 32*, 2332–40.

Adler, A. (1921). *The Neurotic Constitution: Outlines of a Comparative Individualistic Psychology* (translated from the German). London: Routledge.

American Psychiatric Association (1980). *Diagnostic and Statistical Manual of Mental Disorders, Third Edition* (DSM-III). Washington, DC: American Psychiatric Association.

Andrews, G. (1996). Comorbidity and the general neurotic syndrome. *British Journal of Psychiatry, 168* (Supplement 30), 76–84.

Andrews, G., Stewart, G., Morris-Yates, A., Holt, P. & Henderson, S. (1990). Evidence for a general neurotic syndrome. *British Journal of Psychiatry, 157*, 6–12.

Andrews, G., Hobbs, M. J., Borkovec, T. D. et al. (2010). Generalised worry disorder: a review of DSM-IV generalised anxiety disorder and options for DSM-V. *Depression and Anxiety, 27*, 134–47.

Anjara, S. G., Bonetto, C., Ganguli, P. et al. (2019). Can general practitioners manage mental disorders in primary care? A partially randomised, pragmatic, cluster trial. *PLoS One, 14*, e0224724.

Aronson, T. A. (1987). Is panic disorder a distinct diagnostic entity? A critical review of the borders of a syndrome. *Journal of Nervous and Mental Diseases, 175*, 584–94.

Åsberg, M., Montgomery, S. A., Perris, C., Schalling, D. & Sedvall, G. (1978). A comprehensive psychopathological rating scale. *Acta Psychiatrica Scandinavica* (Supplement), *271*, 5–27.

Balint, M. (1964). *The Doctor, His Patient and the Illness*. London: Pitman.

Barrett, J. E., Barrett, J. A., Oxman, T. E. & Gerber, P. D. (1988). The prevalence of psychiatric disorders in a primary care practice. *Archives of General Psychiatry, 45*, 1100–6.

Bayer, R. & Spitzer, R. L. (1985). Neurosis, psychodynamics, and DSM-III: a history of the controversy. *Archives of General Psychiatry 1985, 42*, 187–96.

Berk, M., Boyce, P., Hamilton, A. et al. (2018). Personality: distraction or driver in the diagnosis of depression. *Personality and Mental Health, 12*, 126–30.

Bernreuter, R. G. (1931). *The Personality Inventory*. Palo Alto, CA: Consulting Psychologists Press.

Bond, M. & Perry, J. C. (2006). Psychotropic medication use, personality disorder and improvement in long-term dynamic psychotherapy. *Journal of Nervous and Mental Disease, 194*, 21–6.

Boyd, J. H., Burke, J. D., Jr, Gruenberg, E. et al. (1984). Exclusion criteria of DSM-III: a study of co-occurrence of hierarchy-free syndromes. *Archives of General Psychiatry, 41*, 983–9.

Brothwell, J., Casey, P. R. & Tyrer, P. (1992). Who gives the most reliable account of a psychiatric patient's personality? *Irish Journal of Psychological Medicine, 9*, 90–3.

Carr, V. J. & Donovan, P. (1992). Psychiatry in general practice: a pilot scheme using the liaison-attachment model. *Medical Journal of Australia, 156*, 379–82.

Casey, P. (2018). *Adjustment Disorders: From Controversy to Clinical Practice*. Oxford: Oxford University Press.

Casey, P. R. & Tyrer, P. J. (1986). Personality, functioning and symptomatology. *Journal of Psychiatric Research, 20*, 363–74.

Casey, P. R., Tyrer, P. J. & Platt, S. (1985). The relationship between social functioning and psychiatric symptomatology in primary care. *Social Psychiatry, 20*, 5–9.

Cattell, R. B. & Stice, G. E. (1957). *The Sixteen Personality Factors Questionnaire*. Champaign, IL: Institute for Personality and Ability Testing.

Cavallaro, R., Regazzetti, M. G., Mundo, E., Brancato, V. & Smeraldi, E. (1993). Tardive dyskinesia outcomes: clinical and pharmacologic correlates of remission and persistence. *Neuropsychopharmacology, 8*, 233–9.

Conan Doyle, A. (1892). *The Adventure of Silver Blaze*. London: Strand Magazine.

Coryell, W., Endicott, J., Andreasen, N. C. et al. (1988). Depression and panic attacks: the significance of overlap as reflected in follow-up and family study data. *American Journal of Psychiatry, 145*, 293–300.

Costa, P. T. & McCrae, R. R. (1992). *Revised NEO Personality Inventory (NEO-PI-R) and NEO Five-Factor Inventory (NEO-FFI) Manual*. Odessa, FL: Psychological Assessment Resources.

Craske, M. G. & Stein, M. B. (2016). Anxiety. *Lancet, 388*, 3048–59.

Cuesta, M. J., Gil, P., Artamendi, M., Serrano, J. F. & Peralta, V. (2002). Premorbid personality and psychopathological dimensions in first-episode psychosis. *Schizophrenia Research, 58*, 273–80.

Cullen, W. (1777). *First Lines of The Practice of Physic*. Edinburgh: Creech.

Darling, C. & Tyrer, P. (1990). Brief encounters in general practice: an audit of liaison in general practice psychiatric clinics. *Psychiatric Bulletin, 14*, 592–4.

Das Munshi, J., Goldberg, D., Bebbington, P. E. et al. (2008). Public health significance of mixed anxiety and depression: beyond current classification. *British Journal of Psychiatry, 192*, 171–7.

Dobson, K. S. (1985). The relationship between anxiety and depression. *Clinical Psychology Review, 5*, 307–24.

Doll, R. & Hill, A. B. (1954). The mortality of doctors in relation to their smoking habits: a preliminary report. *British Medical Journal, 228*, 1451–5.

Doll, R., Peto, R., Wheatley, K., Gray, R. & Sutherland, I. (1994). Mortality in relation to smoking: 40 years' observation on male British doctors. *British Medical Journal, 309*, 901–11.

Duggan, C. F., Lee, A. S. & Murray, R. M. (1990). Does personality predict long-term outcome in depression? *British Journal of Psychiatry, 157*, 19–24.

Duggan, C., Sham, P., Lee, A. & Minne, C. (1996). Neuroticism: a vulnerability marker for depression evidence from a family study. *Journal of Affective Disorders, 35*, 139–43.

Eisenberg, L. (1992). Treating depression and anxiety in primary care: closing the gap between knowledge and practice. *New England Journal of Medicine, 326*, 1080–4.

Emmanuel, J. S., McGee, A., Ukoumunne, O. C. & Tyrer, P. (2002). A randomised controlled trial of enhanced key-worker liaison psychiatry in general practice. *Social Psychiatry and Psychiatric Epidemiology, 37*, 261–6.

Evenden, M., Svanborg, P., Gustavsson, P. & Åsberg, M. (1996). Determinants of self-rating and expert rating concordance in psychiatric out-patients, using the affective subscales of the CPRS. *Acta Psychiatrica Scandinavica, 94*, 386–96.

Eysenck, H. J. (1952). The effects of psychotherapy: an evaluation. *Journal of Consulting and Clinical Psychology, 16*, 319–24.

Feinstein, A. R. (1970). The pre-therapeutic classification of co-morbidity in chronic disease. *Journal of Chronic Diseases, 23*, 455–68.

First, M. B., Spitzer, R. L., Gibbon, M. et al. (1995). The Structured Clinical Interview for DSM-III-R Personality Disorders (SCID-II): II. Multi-site test-retest reliability study. *Journal of Personality Disorders, 9*, 92–104.

Frances, A. (2016). Robert Spitzer: the most influential psychiatrist of his time. *The Lancet Psychiatry, 3*, 110–11.

Fredman, L., Weissman, M. M., Leaf, P. J. & Bruce, M. L. (1988). Social functioning in community residents with depression and other psychiatric disorders: results of the

New Haven Epidemiological Catchment Area study. *Journal of Affective Disorders*, 15, 103–112.

Galen (192 AD). *Mixtures: De Temperamentis*. Ed. and tr. by P. N. Singer, P. J. van der Eijk & P. Tassinari, 2019. Cambridge: Cambridge University Press.

Gask, L., Dowrick, C., Klinkman, M. & Gureje, O. (2018). Diagnosis and classification of mental illness: a view from primary care. In Gask, L., Kendrick, T., Peveler, R. & Chew-Graham, C. A. (eds.), *Primary Care Mental Health*, 2nd ed., pp. 70–85. Cambridge: Cambridge University Press.

Germans, S., Guus L. V. H. & Hodiamont, P.P.G. (2011). Quick Personality Assessment Schedule (PAS-Q): validation of a brief screening test for personality disorders in a population of psychiatric outpatients. *Australian and New Zealand Journal of Psychiatry*, 45, 756–62.

Germans, S., Guus L. V. H. & Hodiamont, P. P. G. (2012). Results of the search for personality disorder screening tools: clinical implications. *Journal of Clinical Psychiatry*, 73, 165–73.

Goldberg, D. (2013). The central importance of anxiety in common mental disorders. *Australian and New Zealand Journal of Psychiatry*, 47, 983–5.

Goldberg, D. & Gater, R. (1991). Estimates of need: a document prepared for the South Manchester District Health Authority. *BJPsych Bulletin*, 15, 593–5.

Goldberg, D. P., Cooper, B., Eastwood, M. R., Kedward, H. B. & Shepherd, M. (1970). A standardized psychiatric interview for use in community surveys. *British Journal of Preventive and Social Medicine*, 24, 18–23.

Grenyer, B. F. S., Lewis, K. L., Fanaian, M. & Kotze, B. (2018). Treatment of personality disorder using a whole of service stepped care approach: a cluster randomized controlled trial. *PLoS ONE 13*, e0206472.

Gurney, C., Roth, M., Garside, R., Kerr, T. & Schapira, K. (1972). Studies in the classification of affective disorders: the relationship between anxiety states and depressive illnesses. II. *British Journal of Psychiatry*, 121, 162–6.

Haddad, P. M. & Nutt, D. J. (eds.). (2020). *Seminars in Clinical Psychopharmacology*, 3rd ed. Oxford: Oxford University Press.

Hathaway, S. R. & McKinley, J. C. (1940). A multiphasic personality schedule (Minnesota): I. Construction of the schedule. *Journal of Psychology*, 10, 249–54.

Henderson, D. K. & Batchelor, I. R. C. (1969). *Henderson and Gillespie's Textbook of Psychiatry*, 10th ed. Oxford: Oxford University Press.

Herrmann, N., Black, S. E., Lawrence, J., Szekely, C. & Szalai, J. P. (1998). The Sunnybrook Stroke Study: a prospective study of depressive symptoms and functional outcome. *Stroke, 29*, 618–24.

Hettema, J. M., Neale, M. C. & Kendler, K. S. (2001). A review and meta-analysis of the genetic epidemiology of anxiety disorders. *American Journal of Psychiatry, 158*, 1568–78.

Hill, J., Fudge, H., Harrington, R., Pickles, A. & Rutter, M. (2000). Complementary approaches to the assessment of personality disorder. *British Journal of Psychiatry, 176*, 434–9.

Jackson, G., Gater, R., Goldberg, D., Tantam, D., Loftus, L. & Taylor. H. (1993). A new community mental health team based in primary care: a description of the service and its effect on service use in the first year. *British Journal of Psychiatry, 162*, 375–84.

Kendell, R. (1975a). *The Role of Diagnosis in Psychiatry*. London: Blackwell.

Kendell, R. (1975b). The concept of disease and its implications for psychiatry. *British Journal of Psychiatry, 127*, 305–15.

Kendell, R. E. (1991). The major functional psychoses: are they independent entities or part of a continuum? In Kerr, A. & McClelland, H. *Concepts of Mental Illness: A Continuing Debate*, pp. 1–16. London: Gaskell.

Kendell, R. E. & Jablensky, A. (2003). Distinguishing between the validity and utility of psychiatric diagnoses. *American Journal of Psychiatry, 160*, 4–12.

Kendell, R. E., Cooper, J. E., Gourlay, A. J., Copeland, J. R. M., Sharpe, L. & Gurland, B. J. (1971). Diagnostic criteria of American and

British psychiatrists. *Archives of General Psychiatry*, 25, 123–30.

Kerr, T. A., Roth, M., Schapira, K. & Gurney, C. (1972). The assessment and prediction of outcome in affective disorders. *British Journal of Psychiatry*, 121, 167–74.

Kiloh, L. G., Andrews, G., Neilson, M. & Bianchi, G. (1972). The relationship of the syndromes called endogenous and neurotic depression. *British Journal of Psychiatry*, 121, 183–96.

Kingdon, D., Tyrer, P., Seivewright, N., Ferguson, B. & Murphy, S. (1996). The Nottingham Study of Neurotic Disorder: influence of cognitive therapists on outcome. *British Journal of Psychiatry*, 169, 93–7.

Klein, D. F. (1964). Delineation of two drug-responsive anxiety syndromes. *Psychopharmacologia*, 5, 397–408.

Klein, D. F. (1981). Anxiety Reconceptualized. In Klein, D. F. & Rabkin, J. G. (eds.), *Anxiety: New Research and Changing Concepts*, pp. 235–62. New York: Raven Press.

Klein, D. F. (1988). Nottingham Study of Neurotic Disorder. *Lancet*, 332, 1015.

Knerer, G., Byford, S., Johnson, T., Seivewright, H. & Tyrer, P. (2005). The Nottingham Study of Neurotic Disorder: predictors of 12 years costs. *Acta Psychiatrica Scandinavica*, 112, 224–32.

Lahey, B. B. (2009). Public health significance of neuroticism. *American Psychologist*, 64, 241–56.

Lancet (editorial) (1959). The nature of essential hypertension. *Lancet*, 274, 895–6.

Lewis, G. (1991). Observer bias and the assessment of anxiety and depression. *Social Psychiatry and Psychiatric Epidemiology*, 26, 265–72.

Lewis, G. (1992). Measuring psychiatric disorder in the community: a standardized assessment for use by lay interviewers. *Psychological Medicine*, 22, 465–86.

Lilienfeld, S. O., Lynn, S. J., Ruscio, J. & Beyerstein, B. L. (2009). *50 Great Myths of Popular Psychology: Shattering Widespread Misconceptions about Human Behavior*. Chichester: Wiley-Blackwell.

McHugh, K., Swamy, G. K. & Hernandez, A. F. (2018). Engaging patients throughout the health system: a landscape analysis of cold-call policies and recommendations for future policy change. *Journal of Clinical and Translational Science*, 6, 384–92.

Meyer, A. (1902). *Collected Papers*, 2, 90–104. Baltimore, MD: Johns Hopkins Press.

Mindham, R. H. S. (2020). Mapperley Hospital, Nottingham and George Hine: a creative relationship. *British Journal of Psychiatry*, 216, 174.

Mitchell, A. J., Meader, N. & Symonds, P. (2010). Diagnostic validity of the Hospital Anxiety and Depression Scale (HADS) in cancer and palliative settings: a meta-analysis. *Journal of Affective Disorders*, 126, 335–48.

Montgomery, S. A. & Åsberg, M. (1979). A new depression scale designed to be sensitive to change. *British Journal of Psychiatry*, 134, 382–9.

Morrison, H. (2016). Constructing patient stories: 'dynamic' case notes and clinical encounters at Glasgow's Gartnavel Mental Hospital, 1921–32. *Medical History*, 60, 67–86.

Mundt, J. C., Marks, I. M., Shear, M. K. & Greist, J. H. (2002). The Work and Social Adjustment Scale: a simple measure of impairment in functioning. *British Journal of Psychiatry*, 180, 461–4

Murphy, S. M., Owen, R. T. & Tyrer, P. J. (1984). Withdrawal symptoms after six weeks treatment with diazepam. *Lancet*, 324, 1389.

Murray, H. A. (1943). *Manual for the Thematic Appreciation Test*. Cambridge, MA: Harvard University Press.

Newton-Howes, G., Tyrer, P., Johnson, T. et al. (2014). Influence of personality on the outcome of treatment in depression: systematic review and meta-analysis. *Journal of Personality Disorders*, 28, 577–93.

Oldham, P. D., Pickering, G., Fraser Roberts, J. A. & Sowry, G. S. C. (1960). The nature of essential hypertension. *Lancet*, 275, 1085–93.

Pappworth, M. (1971). *A Primer of Medicine*. London: Butterworth.

Paykel, E. S. (2008). Basic concepts of depression. *Dialogues in Clinical Neuroscience, 10*, 279–89.

Pickering, G. (1960). The nature of essential hypertension. *Lancet, 275*, 170.

Piñero, J. M. L. (1983). *Historical Origins of the Concept of Neurosis.* Cambridge: Cambridge University Press.

Platt, R. (1959). The nature of essential hypertension. *Lancet, 274*, 1092.

Plomin, R. (2011). Commentary: Why are children in the same family so different? Non-shared environment three decades later. *International Journal of Epidemiology, 40*, 582–92.

Plomin, R. & Daniels, D. (1987). Why are children in the same family so different from each other? *Behavioural and Brain Sciences, 10*, 1–16.

Quinton, D., Gulliver, L. & Rutter, M. (1995). A 15–20 year follow-up of adult psychiatric patients: psychiatric disorder and social functioning. *British Journal of Psychiatry, 167*, 315–23.

Remington, M. & Tyrer, P. (1979). The Social Functioning Schedule: a brief semi-structured interview. *Social Psychiatry, 14*, 151–7

Rorschach, H. (1921). *Psychodiagnostik.* Bern: Hans Huber.

Rosenhan, D. L. (1973). On being sane in insane places. *Science, 179*, 250–8.

Roth, M., Gurney, C., Garside, R. F. & Kerr, T. A (1972). Studies in the classification of affective disorders: the relationship between anxiety states and depressive illnesses. *British Journal of Psychiatry, 121*, 147–61.

Sanatinia, R., Afzal, S., MacLaren, T. et al. (2019). Improved mental health among LABILE study participants: a qualitative exploration. *Personality and Mental Health, 13*, 75–83.

Schapira, K., Roth, M., Kerr, T. A. & Gurney, C. (1972). The prognosis of affective disorders: the differentiation of anxiety states from depressive illnesses. *British Journal of Psychiatry, 121*, 175–81.

Seivewright, H., Tyrer, P. & Johnson, T. (1998). Prediction of outcome in neurotic disorder: a five-year prospective study. *Psychological Medicine, 28*, 1149–57.

Seivewright, H., Tyrer, P. & Johnson, T. (2004). Persistent social dysfunction in anxious and depressed patients with personality disorder. *Acta Psychiatrica Scandinavica, 109*, 104–9.

Snaith, P. (1991). *Clinical Neurosis.* Oxford: Oxford University Press.

Spiegel, A. (2005). The dictionary of disorder: how one man revolutionized psychiatry. *New Yorker*, January 3.

Spitzer, R. L. & Williams, J. B. (1983). *Structured Clinical Interview for DSM-III (1983 version).* New York: New York State Psychiatric Institute.

Spitzer, R. L. & Wilson, P. T. (1968). *American Psychiatric Association, Diagnostic and Statistical Manual of Mental Disorders: 2.* Washington, DC: American Psychiatric Association.

Stern, A. F. (2014). The Hospital Anxiety and Depression Scale. *Occupational Medicine, 64*, 393–4.

Surtees, P. G. & Barkley, C. (1994). Future imperfect: the long-term outcome of depressive disorder. *British Journal of Psychiatry, 164*, 327–41.

Thompson, C., Kinmonth, A. L., Stevens, L. et al. (2000). Effects of a clinical-practice guideline and practice-based education on detection and outcome of depression in primary care: Hampshire Depression Project randomised controlled trial. *Lancet, 355*, 185–91.

Thompson, F. (1887). In No Strange Land, from *The works of Francis Thompson.* Leopold Classic Library, 2015

Tyrer, P. (1985). Neurosis divisible? *Lancet, 325*, 685–88.

Tyrer, P. (1989). *Classification of Neurosis.* Chichester: John Wiley.

Tyrer, P. (1991). Neuroses and personality disorders. In Kerr. A. & McClelland, H. (eds.), *Concepts of Mental Disorder*, pp. 112–28. London: Gaskell.

Tyrer, P. (1996). Comorbidity or consanguinity. *British Journal of Psychiatry, 168*, 669–71.

Tyrer, P. (2007). Personality diatheses: a superior explanation than disorder. *Psychological Medicine*, 37, 1521–5.

Tyrer, P. (2008a). The whys and wares of the yellow vans. From the Editor's Desk. *British Journal of Psychiatry*, 193, 350.

Tyrer, P. (2008b). So careless of the single trial. *Evidence-Based Mental Health*, 11, 65–6.

Tyrer, P. (2009). *Nidotherapy: Harmonising the Environment with the Patient*. London: RCPsych Publications.

Tyrer, P. (2013). The swings and roundabouts of community mental health: the UK fairground. In Thornicroft, G., Ruggeri, M. & Goldberg, D. (eds.), *Improving Mental Health Care: The Global Challenge*, pp. 25–40. Chichester: Wiley-Blackwell.

Tyrer, P. (2021). *Overcoming personality disorder: it's in your hands*. Lincoln: Impspired.

Tyrer, P. & Alexander, J. (1979). Classification of personality disorder. *British Journal of Psychiatry*, 135, 163–7.

Tyrer, P. & Casey, P. (1993). *Social Function in Psychiatry: The Hidden Axis of Classification Exposed*. Petersfield: Wrightson Biomedical Publishing.

Tyrer, P. & Johnson, T. (1996). Establishing the severity of personality disorder. *American Journal of Psychiatry*, 153, 1593–7.

Tyrer, P. & Remington, M. (1979). Controlled comparison of day hospital and outpatient treatment for neurotic disorders. *Lancet*, 313, 1014–16.

Tyrer, P., Casey, P. & Gall, J. (1983). The relationship between neurosis and personality disorder. *British Journal of Psychiatry*, 142, 404–408.

Tyrer, P., Ferguson, B. & Wadsworth, J. (1990). Liaison psychiatry in general practice: the comprehensive collaborative model. *Acta Psychiatrica Scandinavica*, 81, 359–63.

Tyrer, P., Owen, R. T. & Cicchetti, D. V. (1984). The brief scale for anxiety: a subdivision of the Comprehensive Psychopathological Rating Scale. *Journal of Neurology, Neurosurgery and Psychiatry*, 47, 970–5.

Tyrer, P., Turner, R. & Johnson, A. L. (1989). Integrated hospital and community psychiatric services and use of inpatient beds. *British Medical Journal*, 299, 298–300.

Tyrer, P., Tyrer, H. & Yang, M. (2021). Premature mortality of people with personality disorder in the Nottingham Study of Neurotic Disorder. *Personality and Mental Health*, 15, 32–39.

Tyrer, P., Tyrer, H. & Yang, M. (2022). Treatments received in the Nottingham Study of Neurotic Disorder over 30 years: comparison of groups by personality status. *Personality and Mental Health*, January. https://doi.org/10.1002/pmh .1535.

Tyrer, P., Alexander, J., Remington, M. & Riley, P. (1987). Relationship between neurotic symptoms and neurotic diagnosis: a longitudinal study. *Journal of Affective Disorders*, 13, 13–21.

Tyrer, P., Mitchard, S., Methuen, C. & Ranger, M. (2003). Treatment-rejecting and treatment-seeking personality disorders: Type R and Type S. *Journal of Personality Disorders*, 17, 265–70.

Tyrer, P., Mulder, R., Kim, Y-R. & Crawford, M. J. (2019). The development of the ICD-11 classification of personality disorders: an amalgam of science, pragmatism and politics. *Annual Review of Clinical Psychology*, 15, 481–502.

Tyrer, P., Seivewright, H., Ferguson, B. & Johnson, T. (2003). 'Cold calling' in psychiatric follow-up studies: is it justified? *Journal of Medical Ethics*, 29, 238–42.

Tyrer, P., Seivewright, N., Ferguson, B. & Tyrer, J. (1992). The general neurotic syndrome: a coaxial diagnosis of anxiety, depression and personality disorder. *Acta Psychiatrica Scandinavica*, 85, 201–6.

Tyrer, P., Yang, M., Tyrer, H. & Crawford, M. (2021). Is social function a good proxy measure of personality disorder? *Personality and Mental Health*, 15, 261–72.

Tyrer, P., Alexander, M. S., Cicchetti, D., Cohen, M. S. & Remington, M. (1979). Reliability of a schedule for rating personality disorders. *British Journal of Psychiatry*, 135, 168–74.

Tyrer, P., Nur, U., Crawford, M., Karlsen, S., McLean, C., Rao, B., & Johnson, T. (2005). The Social Functioning Questionnaire: a rapid and robust measure of perceived functioning. *International Journal of Social Psychiatry*, *51*, 265–75.

Tyrer, P., Seivewright, N., Ferguson, B., Murphy, S. & Johnson, A. L. (1993). The Nottingham study of neurotic disorder: impact of personality status on response to drug treatment, cognitive therapy and self-help over two years. *British Journal of Psychiatry*, *162*, 219–26.

Tyrer, P., Seivewright, N., Ferguson, B. et al. (1988). Nottingham Study of Neurotic Disorder. *Lancet*, *332*, 1015.

Tyrer, P., Seivewright, N., Murphy, S. et al. (1988). The Nottingham Study of Neurotic Disorder: comparison of drug and psychological treatments. *Lancet*, *332*, 235–40.

Tyrer, P., Seivewright, N, Ferguson, B. et al. (1990). The Nottingham Study of Neurotic Disorder: relationship between personality status and symptoms. *Psychological Medicine*, *20*, 423–31.

Tyrer, P., Crawford, M., Sanatinia, R. et al. (2014). Preliminary studies of the ICD-11 classification of personality disorder in practice. *Personality and Mental Health*, *8*, 254–63.

Whytt, R. (1765). *Observations on the Nature, Causes and Cure of Those Disorders Which Have Commonly Been Called, Nervous Hypochondriac or Hysteric*. Edinburgh: J. Balfour.

Williams, P. & Balestrieri, M. (1989). Psychiatric clinics in general practice: do they reduce admissions? *British Journal of Psychiatry*, *154*, 67–71.

World Health Organisation (2018). *ICD-11, the 11th Revision of the International Classification of Diseases* [Online]. Geneva: World Health Organisation. https://icd.who.int/ [accessed 21 January 2021].

Yang, M., Tyrer, P. & Tyrer, H. (2022). The recording of personality strengths: an analysis of the impact of positive personality features on the long-term outcome of common mental disorders. *Personality and Mental Health* (in press).

Yang, M., Tyrer, H., Johnson, T. & Tyrer, P. (2022). Personality change in the Nottingham Study of Neurotic Disorder: 30 year cohort study. *Australian and New Zealand Journal of Psychiatry*, *56*, 260–9.

Zigmond, A. S. & Snaith, R. P. (1983). The Hospital Anxiety and Depression Scale. *Acta Psychiatrica Scandinavica*, *57*, 361–70.

Index